HEALTH AND HUMAN DEVELOPMENT

HUMAN IMMUNODEFICIENCY VIRUS (HIV) RESEARCH

SOCIAL SCIENCE ASPECTS

HEALTH AND HUMAN DEVELOPMENT

JOAV MERRICK - SERIES EDITOR –

HEALTH SERVICES, DIVISION FOR INTELLECTUAL
AND DEVELOPMENTAL DISABILITIES
MINISTRY OF SOCIAL AFFAIRS, JERUSALEM, ISRAEL

Adolescent Behavior Research: International Perspectives
Joav Merrick and Hatim A. Omar (Editors)
2007. ISBN: 1-60021-649-8

Complementary Medicine Systems: Comparison and Integration
Karl W. Kratky
2008. ISBN: 978-1-60456-475-4 (Hardcover)
2008. ISBN: 978-1-61122-433-7 (E-book)

Pain in Children and Youth
Patricia Schofield and Joav Merrick (Editors)
2008. ISBN: 978-1-60456-951-3

Challenges in Adolescent Health: An Australian Perspective
David Bennett, Susan Towns, Elizabeth Elliott and Joav Merrick (Editors)
2009. ISBN: 978-1-60741-616-6 (Hardcover)
2009. ISBN: 978-1-61668-240-8 (E-book)

Behavioral Pediatrics, 3rd Edition
Donald E. Greydanus, Dilip R. Patel, Helen D. Pratt and Joseph L. Calles, Jr. (Editors)
2009. ISBN: 978-1-60692-702-1 (Hardcover)
2009. ISBN: 978-1-60876-630-7 (E-book)

Health and Happiness from Meaningful Work: Research in Quality of Working Life
Søren Ventegodt and Joav Merrick (Editors)
2009. ISBN: 978-1-60692-820-2

Obesity and Adolescence: A Public Health Concern
Hatim A. Omar, Donald E. Greydanus, Dilip R. Patel and Joav Merrick (Editors)
2009. ISBN: 978-1-60456-821-9

Poverty and Children: A Public Health Concern
Alexis Lieberman and Joav Merrick (Editors)
2009. ISBN: 978-1-60741-140-6

Living on the Edge: The Mythical, Spiritual, and Philosophical Roots of Social Marginality
Joseph Goodbread
2009. ISBN: 978-1-60741-162-8

Alcohol-Related Cognitive Disorders: Research and Clinical Perspectives
Leo Sher, Isack Kandel and Joav Merrick (Editors)
2009. ISBN: 978-1-60741-730-9 (Hardcover)
2009. ISBN: 978-1-60876-623-9 (E-book)

Rural Child Health: International Aspects
Erica Bell and Joav Merrick (Editors)
2010. ISBN: 978-1-60876-357-3 (Hardcover)
2010. ISBN: 978-1-61324-005-2 (E-book)

Children and Pain
Patricia Schofield and Joav Merrick (Editors)
2009. ISBN: 978-1-60876-020-6 (Hardcover)
2009. ISBN: 978-1-61728-183-9 (E-book)

Conceptualizing Behavior in Health and Social Research: A Practical Guide to Data Analysis
Said Shahtahmasebi and Damon Berridge
2010. ISBN: 978-1-60876-383-2

Chance Action and Therapy: The Playful Way of Changing
Uri Wernik
2010. ISBN: 978-1-60876-393-1 (Hardcover)
2011. ISBN: 978-1-61122-987-5 (Softcover)
2011. ISBN: 978-1-61209-874-6 (E-book)

Adolescence and Chronic Illness. A Public Health Concern
Hatim Omar, Donald E. Greydanus, Dilip R. Patel and Joav Merrick (Editors)
2010. ISBN: 978-1-60876-628-4 (Hardcover)
2010. ISBN: 978-1-61761-482-8 (E-book)

Adolescence and Sports
Dilip R. Patel, Donald E. Greydanus, Hatim Omar and Joav Merrick (Editors)
2010. ISBN: 978-1-60876-702-1 (Hardcover)
2010. ISBN: 978-1-61761-483-5 (E-book)

International Aspects of Child Abuse and Neglect
Howard Dubowitz and Joav Merrick (Editors)
2010. ISBN: 978-1-60876-703-8 (Hardcover)
2010. ISBN: 978-1-61122-049-0 (Softcover)
2010. ISBN: 978-1-61122-403-0 (E-book)

Positive Youth Development: Evaluation and Future Directions in a Chinese Context
Daniel T.L. Shek, Hing Keung Ma and Joav Merrick (Editors)
2010. ISBN: 978-1-60876-830-1 (Hardcover)
2010. ISBN: 978-1-61668-376-4 (E-book)
2011. ISBN: 978-1-62100-175-1 (Softcover)

Positive Youth Development: Implementation of a Youth Program in a Chinese Context
Daniel T.L Shek, Hing Keung Ma and Joav Merrick (Editors)
2010. ISBN: 978-1-61668-230-9 (Hardcover)
2010. ISBN: 978-1-61209-091-7 (E-book)

Pediatric and Adolescent Sexuality and Gynecology: Principles for the Primary Care Clinician
Hatim A. Omar, Donald E. Greydanus, Artemis K. Tsitsika, Dilip R. Patel and Joav Merrick (Editors)
2010. ISBN: 978-1-60876-735-9

Understanding Eating Disorders: Integrating Culture, Psychology and Biology
Yael Latzer, Joav Merrick and Daniel Stein (Editors)
2011. ISBN: 978-1-61728-298-0 (Hardcover)
2011. ISBN: 978-1-61470- 976-3 (Softcover)
2011. ISBN: 978-1-61942-054-0 (E-book)

Advanced Cancer Pain and Quality of Life
Edward Chow and Joav Merrick (Editors)
2010. ISBN: 978-1-61668-207-1 (Hardcover)
2010. ISBN: 978-1-61668-400-6 (E-book)

Bone and Brain Metastases: Advances in Research and Treatment
Arjun Sahgal, Edward Chow and Joav Merrick (Editors)
2010. ISBN: 978-1-61668-365-8 (Hardcover)
2010. ISBN: 978-1-61728-085-6 (E-book)

Environment, Mood Disorders and Suicide
Teodor T. Postolache and Joav Merrick (Editors)
2010. ISBN: 978-1-61668-505-8

Social and Cultural Psychiatry Experience from the Caribbean Region
Hari D. Maharajh and Joav Merrick (Editors)
2010. ISBN: 978-1-61668-506-5 (Hardcover)
2010. ISBN: 978-1-61728-088-7 (E-book)

Narratives and Meanings of Migration
Julia Mirsky
2010. ISBN: 978-1-61761-103-2 (Hardcover)
2010. ISBN: 978-1-61761-519-1 (E-book)

Self-Management and the Health Care Consumer
Peter William Harvey
2011. ISBN: 978-1-61761-796-6 (Hardcover)
2011. ISBN: 978-1-61122-214-2 (E-book)

Sexology from a Holistic Point of View
Soren Ventegodt and Joav Merrick
2011. ISBN: 978-1-61761-859-8 (Hardcover)
2011. ISBN: 978-1-61122-262-3 (E-book)

Principles of Holistic Psychiatry: A Textbook on Holistic Medicine for Mental Disorders
Soren Ventegodt and Joav Merrick
2011. ISBN: 978-1-61761-940-3 (Hardcover)
2011. ISBN: 978-1-61122-263-0 (E-book)

Clinical Aspects of Psychopharmacology in Childhood and Adolescence
Donald E. Greydanus, Joseph L. Calles, Jr., Dilip P. Patel, Ahsan Nazeer and Joav Merrick (Editors)
2011. ISBN: 978-1-61122-135-0 (Hardcover)
2011. ISBN: 978-1-61122-715-4 (E-book)

Climate Change and Rural Child Health
Erica Bell, Bastian M. Seidel and Joav Merrick (Editors)
2011. ISBN: 978-1-61122-640-9 (Hardcover)
2011. ISBN: 978-1-61209-014-6 (E-book)

Rural Medical Education: Practical Strategies
Erica Bell, Craig Zimitat and Joav Merrick (Editors)
2011. ISBN: 978-1-61122-649-2 (Hardcover)

Advances in Environmental Health Effects of Toxigenic Mold and Mycotoxins
Ebere Cyril Anyanwu
2011. ISBN: 978-1-60741-953-2

Child and Adolescent Health Yearbook 2009
Joav Merrick
2011. ISBN: 978-1-61668-913-1 (Hardcover)

Public Health Yearbook 2009
Joav Merrick
2011. ISBN: 978-1-61668-911-7 (Hardcover)

Child Health and Human Development Yearbook 2009
Joav Merrick
2011. ISBN: 978-1-61668-912-4 (Hardcover)

Alternative Medicine Yearbook 2009
Joav Merrick (Editor)
2011. ISBN: 978-1-61668-910-0 (Hardcover)

The Dance of Sleeping and Eating among Adolescents: Normal and Pathological Perspectives
Yael Latzer and Orna Tzischinsky (Editors)
2011. ISBN: 978-1-61209-710-7 (Hardcover)

Child and Adolescent Health Yearbook 2010
Joav Merrick (Editor)
2011. ISBN: 978-1-61209-788-6 (Hardcover)

Child Health and Human Development Yearbook 2010
Joav Merrick (Editor)
2011. ISBN: 978-1-61209-789-3

Public Health Yearbook 2010
Joav Merrick (Editor)
2011. ISBN: 978-1-61209-971-2

Living on the Edge: The Mythical, Spiritual, and Philosophical Roots of Social Marginality
Joseph Goodbread (Editor)
2011. ISBN: 978-1-60741-162-8 (Hardcover)
2011. ISBN: 978-1-61122-986-8 (Softcover)

Alternative Medicine Yearbook 2010
Joav Merrick (Editor)
2011. ISBN: 978-1-62100-132-4 (Hardcover)
2011. ISBN: 978-1-62100-210-9 (E-book)

The Astonishing Brain and Holistic Conciousness: Neuroscience and Vedanta Perspectives
Vinod D. Deshmukh
2011. ISBN: 978-1-61324-295-7 (Hardcover)

Translational Research for Primary Healthcare
Erica Bell and Joav Merrick (Editors)
2011. ISBN: 978-1-61324-647-4 (Hardcover)

Drug Abuse in Hong Kong: Development and Evaluation of a Prevention Program
Daniel T.L. Shek, Rachel C.F. Sun and Joav Merrick (Editors)
2011. ISBN: 978-1-61324-491-3 (Hardcover)

Human Development: Biology from a Holistic Point of View
Søren Ventegodt, Tyge Dahl Hermansen and Joav Merrick (Editors)
2011. ISBN: 978-1-61470-441-6 (Hardcover)
2011. ISBN: 978-1-61470-541-3 (E-book)

Our Search for Meaning in Life
Søren Ventegodt and Joav Merrick (Editors)
2011. ISBN: 978-1-61470-494-2 (Hardcover)
2011. ISBN: 978-1-61470-519-2 (E-book)

HEALTH AND HUMAN DEVELOPMENT

HUMAN IMMUNODEFICIENCY VIRUS (HIV) RESEARCH

SOCIAL SCIENCE ASPECTS

HUGH KLEIN
AND
JOAV MERRICK
EDITORS

Nova Biomedical Books
New York

For permission to use material from this book please contact us:
Telephone 631-231-7269; Fax 631-231-8175
Web Site: http://www.novapublishers.com

Library of Congress Cataloging-in-Publication Data

ISBN 978-1-62081-293-8

Library of Congress Control Number: 2012933664

Published by Nova Science Publishers, Inc. † New York

Contents

Preface

Looking back over the course of the three-plus decades of the HIV/AIDS epidemic, scholars and researchers have made many significant strides in understanding and responding to HIV and AIDS. From the inception of the HIV/AIDS epidemic during the early 1980s until the mid-1990s, when highly active antiretroviral treatment (HAART) was introduced as an innovative and highly-effective way of controlling HIV and HIV-related diseases, the "average" person diagnosed as being HIV-positive could expect to live for several months and if lucky, for a few years. Today, with the medical advances that have been made in the fight against HIV/AIDS, people who have contracted HIV usually can expect to live relatively healthy lives, in most instances for many years without experiencing any serious complications of HIV disease. This book focuses on the social science aspects of current HIV research.

Chapter I – Self-report measures of condom use are frequently used to determine the efficacy of HIV prevention programs, however, little is known about which condom use formats yield the most reliable data. The authors' study was conducted to determine how often adolescents respond reliably across three formats of condom use (dichotomous, ordinal, and continuous) and whether participant characteristics are associated with inconsistency. Survey data were collected from 1,190 adolescents, 15-21 years, participating in a behavioral HIV-prevention trial. Approximately 40% were inconsistent in their reports of condom use. Participant characteristics were not associated with consistency in responding. The authors conclude that single items of condom use may suffice for some purposes, but more precise measurement may require multiple formats.

Chapter II – HIV-specific statutes are increasingly popular in the United States and often impose harsh penalties for failure to disclose an HIV diagnosis to sexual partners. The purpose of this study was to examine HIV-related websites for information about non-disclosure as a crime and the relevance of this advice for US audiences. Internet searches were conducted for HIV-related websites with advice on disclosure to sexual partners. Once identified, these sites were analyzed for content, quality, and type of approach to disclosure and the law. Each site was given a page ranking (P. Score) according to Google's priority listing algorithm, and a value ranking (V. Score) for textual content and quality of advice. Internet advice on disclosure and the law was highly variable. With few exceptions, highly ranked US sites offered less advice than sites in Britain, Canada and Australia. All US sites followed the law by placing the onus of responsibility for disclosure on the HIV-infected individual but few offered advice on how to disclose or how to obtain proof of disclosure in order to avoid prosecution. None addressed the special risks of African Americans who are most likely to be prosecuted for non-disclosure. It is concluded that HIV advice websites should offer strategies on how to disclose to sexual partners and to document proof in case of prosecution.

Chapter III – Using a Syndemics Theory conceptual model, this study examines the relationship between childhood maltreatment experiences and involvement in HIV risk taking in a sample of adult men who actively seek partners for unprotected sex via the Internet. The study was based on a national random sample of 332 men who have sex with men (MSM), who use the Internet to seek men with whom they can engage in unprotected sex. Data collection was conducted via telephone interviews between January 2008 and May 2009. Structural equation analysis was undertaken to examine the specific nature of the relationships involved in understanding HIV risk practices. Childhood maltreatment experiences were not found to be related directly to involvement in HIV risk taking in adulthood. Childhood maltreatment, particularly in the form of emotional neglect, was found to be an important variable in the overall structural equation. Its effect on HIV risk taking was indirect, operating principally by having a negative impact upon self-esteem, which in turn had a negative effect on attitudes toward condom use, which in turn were related strongly and directly to risk taking. The authors conclude that childhood maltreatment experiences are relevant to understanding HIV risk practices among MSM in adulthood, but the relationship is not as simple as usually conceptualized. Rather, childhood maltreatment appears to impact risk taking indirectly, through its effects on mental health functioning, which in turn affects risk-related attitudes.

Chapter IV – Men with a female partner who also have sex with men (MSMW) have been identified as a bridge population for possible HIV transmission to heterosexual women. Social science research that examines how relational and social aspects of MSMW partnered with women is needed to better understand the possible mechanisms that may contribute to HIV/STI risk among MSMW, their female relationship partners, and secondary male sex partners. The authors' study assessed whether self-reported accounts of sexual agreements and relationship behaviors of MSMW with a current female partner corresponded to their sexual risk behaviors with secondary male sex partners. A cross-sectional study design was used to collect anonymous data from a convenience sample of 145 MSMW who had a current female partner and also sought to engage in sex with men. The data indicated that the majority of MSMW engaged in oral and/or anal sex with another male without their female partner knowing. Of men reporting strictly monogamous heterosexual relationships, only 14.5% reported actually only having sex with their female relational partner. The men's average last tests for HIV and STIs were 87.5 and 181.9 months prior, respectively; and most men self-reported low condom use during oral sex and inconsistent condom use during anal intercourse. Universal HIV/STI testing is urgently needed to improve testing rates among MSMW who are unlikely to admit risk-behaviors. Additionally, tailored HIV prevention strategies such as couples-based sexuality and HIV/STI counseling may be beneficial for MSMW.

Chapter V – This chapter explores the stigma experiences of people living with HIV/AIDS (PLWHA) and evaluates the impact of antiretroviral treatment (ART) on their (a) lived experiences and (b) illness management. Qualitative research for this study is based on

105 in-depth interviews and ethnographic observation conducted between May and October of 2008 at an urban HIV clinic in a teaching hospital in Addis Ababa, Ethiopia. A phenomenological approach to data analysis isolated socio-cultural meanings underlying empirical variations of stigma experiences and examined how the availability of treatment alters the experience of living with chronic stigmatized diseases. The study reveals that ART can effect a physical and social rebirth with a renewed sense of self-worth that, together, improve the negative self-concept people develop following an HIV diagnosis. The study also demonstrates that stigma attached to HIV/AIDS remains pervasive in the era of ART. Indeed, ART creates new stigma concerns related to healthcare practices that arise when patients refill prescriptions and follow up on their treatment. This refashioned nature of stigma demands that the authors identify patterns of change in the perception, experience, and management of the illness. Identifying and analyzing sources of stigma for PLWHA allows us to isolate stigma triggers and devise structural changes that can reform elements of healthcare institutions that intensify HIV stigma. Such research is particularly important in resource-poor settings where the AIDS crisis lingers and the socio-cultural factors that influence the outcomes of intervention strategies require attention.

Chapter VI – This chapter examines attitudes toward condom use in a national random sample of 332 MSM who use the Internet to seek men with whom they can engage in unprotected sex. Data collection was conducted via telephone interviews between January 2008 and May 2009. The following three research questions were addressed: 1) How do these men feel about using condoms, both ideologically and personally? 2) How do condom use attitudes relate to actual HIV risk behavior practices? 3) What factors underlie men's attitudes toward condom use? The findings indicated that men held weakly-positive attitudes toward condom use overall, but were noticeably more negative in their attitudes regarding the personal use of condoms. Condom use attitudes were related consistently and inversely to involvement in HIV risk practices. In both multivariate and structural equation analyses, men's condom-related attitudes were the single strongest factor associated with their involvement in risky sex. A number of factors were found to be correlated with more favorable attitudes toward condom use. These were: caring about potential sex partners' HIV serostatus, experiencing fewer drug-related problems, having a lower level of educational attainment, not preferring to have "wild" or "uninhibited" sex, higher self-esteem, being African American, and not perceiving great accuracy in the information that sex partners supply verbally about their HIV serostatus.

Chapter VII – The focus of this chapter is to identify independent correlates of the lack of condom use when engaging in vaginal sex with primary partners among HIV-negative African American adults. The conceptual model includes proximal as well as more distal domains. Cross-sectional data were collected between May 2009 and August 2011. Recruitment involved active and passive recruitment strategies. Computer-assisted, individual interviews were conducted with 1,050 African American adults. Multivariate logistic regression was used to identify independent predictors of a lack of condom use with primary partners in the past 30 days. In multivariate analysis, being older than 35, being partnered, perceiving having a primary partner as important, and ever having been homeless were associated positively with the odds of a lack of condom use during vaginal sex with primary partners in the past 30 days. On the other hand, reporting more than one primary partner in the past 30 days, having health insurance during the past 12 months, and perceived neighborhood social cohesion were negatively associated. These findings highlight the need for HIV risk-reduction prevention and intervention efforts that consider distal as well as proximal domains. Such a perspective allows for a broader sociological inquiry into health disparities that moves beyond epidemiological factors that commonly guide public health research.

In: Human Immunodeficiency Virus …
Editors: Hugh Klein and Joav Merrick

ISBN: 978-1-62081-293-8

Introduction: Social science aspects of current HIV/AIDS research

Hugh Klein*[*1] and Joav Merrick[2,3,4,5]

[1]Kensington Research Institute, Silver Spring, Maryland, US
[2]National Institute of Child Health and Human Development, Jerusalem
[3]Division of Pediatrics, Hadassah Hebrew University Medical Centers, Mt Scopus Campus, Jerusalem
[4]Office of the Medical Director, Health Services, Division for Intellectual and Developmental Disabilities, Ministry of Social Affairs and Social Services, Jerusalem, Israel
[5]Kentucky Children's Hospital, University of Kentucky, Lexington, US

Introduction

Looking back over the course of the three-plus decades of the HIV/AIDS epidemic, scholars and researchers have made many significant strides in understanding and responding to HIV and AIDS. From the inception of the HIV/AIDS epidemic during the early 1980s until the mid-1990s, when highly active antiretroviral treatment (HAART) was introduced as an innovative and highly-effective way of controlling HIV and HIV-related diseases, the "average" person diagnosed as being HIV-positive could expect to live for several months and if lucky, for a few years. Today, with the medical advances that have been made in the fight against HIV/AIDS, people who have contracted HIV usually can expect to live relatively healthy lives, in most instances for many years without experiencing any serious complications of HIV disease. HAART has been so successful that it has resulted in a 94% reduction in excess mortality [1], giving people who have been infected with HIV a significantly longer life and a greatly-lengthened period of healthy living post-infection.

* Correspondence: Hugh Klein, PhD, 401 Schuyler Road, Silver Spring, Maryland 20910 United States. E-mail: hughk@aol.com (primary) and hughkhughk@yahoo.com (secondary)

Research on the exact extent to which HAART adherence reduces the likelihood of sexual transmission of HIV has suggested that the risk of HIV transmission drops by 60-80% when the HIV-infected person adheres to his/her medical regimens and has been taking HAART medications for at least six months [2,3]. Over the course of the three-plus decades of its existence, HIV/AIDS has transitioned from being a short-term death sentence to a long-term manageable condition. In no small part, this transition can be credited to medical and pharmaceutical research advances, which have made strides that, in many ways, are almost miraculous in their scope.

Social science efforts

Simultaneously, while the medical and pharmaceutical researchers were exploring ways to treat HIV-related illnesses and to delay the onset of HIV-related diseases in HIV-infected persons, social science researchers were working to curtail the HIV/AIDS epidemic in other ways. Their efforts focused on different types of research questions, including, among many others such ponderances as these:

- Are all population groups equally at risk for acquiring and/or transmitting HIV? If not, why not?
- Among populations that seem to have a greater risk for acquiring and/or transmitting HIV, what are the factors that lead to their heightened risk?
    - Are these factors psychological or psychosocial in nature, perhaps resulting from having lower self-esteem, greater depression, greater impulsivity, lower perceived self-efficacy, and so forth?
    - Are these factors normative in nature, resulting from societal and/or subcultural expectations pertaining to gender roles, racial/ethnic identities, expressions of sexual identity and sexual orientation, manifestations of masculinity norms, and the like?
    - Are these factors sociocultural in nature, resulting from differences in access to accurate information about HIV transmission based on one's age, gender, race/ethnicity, educational attainment, socioeconomic status, etc?
    - Are these factors socio-structural in nature, resulting from circumstances affecting people's everyday lives and the decisions that they make? This might include romantic partnership or relationship dynamics, previous experiences with childhood trauma, economic necessities that affect how people live their lives, or neighborhood influences on receiving/accepting help from community "outsiders."

- How do various factors co-occur to make the likelihood of HIV acquisition or transmission even greater among some persons–for example, among substance-abusing men who have sex with other men, or among persons who simultaneously are unhappy with their current life circumstances and who see no brighter prospects for their future, or among persons who suffer from the lingering effects of previous abuse and/or neglect and who, as adults, now find themselves involved in a dysfunctional relationship?

Examining these types of questions pertaining to the epidemiology of HIV/AIDS has occupied the time and attention of many hard-working sociologists, psychologists, public health professionals, anthropologists, social workers, and professionals from numerous other disciplines. As a result of their decades of dedicated work, we understand the factors that "drive" the HIV/AIDS epidemic much, much better than we did in years past. Yet there is still much to be learned and understood, particularly about the complex ways in which the multitude of factors that conspire to heighten people's risk for acquiring and/or transmitting HIV interact with one another. In recent years, the emergence of syndemics theory [4,5] and its growing popularity among scholars and researchers in the HIV/AIDS field to understand, predict, and explain involvement in HIV risk-taking [6-9] stands as testament to the complexity of the problems that social scientists face in combating the HIV/AIDS epidemic.

In addition to trying to understand who is at elevated risk for acquiring and/or transmitting HIV and the factors associated with its transmission, social scientists have also devoted a great deal of attention to understanding what is and what is not effective by way of educating people about HIV/AIDS. Developing new and innovative approaches to HIV education, prevention, and intervention, and then evaluating the effectiveness of these various approaches, have been important and ongoing activities among the social scientists and public health professionals working in this field. Learning what works, for whom it works, and under what circumstances it works–and equally importantly, learning what does not work, for whom various approaches are not very effective, and the circumstances that can lead different HIV-related educational, prevention, and intervention efforts to fail, has been the principal goal of public health and social science efforts to curtail the spread of HIV for the past three decades now. Time and again, practitioners have learned the importance of developing culturally-appropriate initiatives to combat HIV [10,11] and the value to be had in developing HIV education, prevention, and intervention programs that are age-appropriate [12,13], gender-specific [14,15], racially/ethnically-sensitive [16,17] and sensitive to the issues pertaining to sexuality and sexual orientation [18,19].

Social aspects

Just as the so-called "bench scientists" continue their critically important work to develop even-more-effective medicines to treat HIV disease and to find a cure for HIV/AIDS, so too do the social scientists continue their efforts to understand the social aspects of HIV and AIDS. Until such time as a cure for AIDS has been identified, our best goals are to learn more about HIV: How it operates inside of the body, how it does the damage that it does to the body's various physiological systems, what specific medications or combinations of medications can be used to slow down or stop the damage that HIV causes to body systems, who (in terms of demographic and/or behavioral trends) is contracting the virus, what the factors are that lead people to engage in transmission-related risk practices, and what can be done to reduce people's inclination to take behavioral risks. Medical and social science researchers alike have played–and continue to play–a critical role in how the HIV/AIDS epidemic unfolds, and medical and social science researchers alike contribute to our ability to keep the negative effects of HIV and AIDS "in check."

The articles included in this special issue of International Public Health Journal represent a small cross-section of some of the types of approaches that contemporary social scientists are taking in their efforts to minimize the harm resulting from HIV and AIDS. These articles represent the utilization of a variety of methodologies, focus on a variety of "at risk" population groups, and advocate a variety of things that might be done from a social science perspective to help curtail the adverse effects of HIV. These articles do not represent social science efforts against HIV as a whole. Rather, they comprise a smattering of different approaches currently underway–a small portion of a much greater whole. Taken as a group, however, they do illustrate one thing quite clearly: Social scientists are working hard to understand HIV and to figure out ways to reduce the harm brought about by HIV infection.

References

[1] Bhaskaran K, Hamouda O, Sannes M, Boufassa F, Johnson AM, Lambert PC, Porter K, CASCADE Collaboration. Changes in the risk of death after HIV seroconversion compared with mortality in the general population. *JAMA* 2008;300:51-9.

[2] Quinn TC, Wawer MJ, Sewnkanbo N, et al. for the Rakai Project Study Group. Viral load and heterosexual transmission of human immunodeficiency virus type-1. *N. Engl. J. Med.* 2000;342:921-9.

[3] Porco TC, Martin JN, Page-Shafer KA, et al. Decline in HIV infectivity following the introduction of highly active antiretroviral therapy. *AIDS* 2004;18:81-8.

[4] Singer M. Introduction to syndemics: A systems approach to public and community health. San Francisco, CA: Jossey-Bass, 2009.

[5] Singer MC, Erickson PI, Badiane L, Diaz R, Ortiz D, Abraham T, Nicolaysen AM. Syndemics, sex and the city: Understanding sexually transmitted diseases in social and cultural context. *Soc. Sci. Med.* 2006;63: 2010-21.

[6] Gielen AC, Ghandour RM, Burke JG, Mahoney P, McDonnell KA, O'Campo P. HIV/AIDS and intimate partner violence: Intersecting women's health issues in the United States. *Trauma Violence Abuse* 2007;8:178-98.

[7] Klein H. Using a syndemics theory approach to study HIV risk taking in a population of men who use the Internet to find partners for unprotected sex. *Am. J. Mens. Health* 2011;5:466-76.

[8] Mustanski B, Garofalo R, Herrick A, Donenberg G. Psychosocial health problems increase risk for HIV among urban young men who have sex with men: Preliminary evidence of a syndemic in need of attention. *Ann. Behav. Med.* 2007;34: 37-45.

[9] Stall R, Friedman M, Cantania JA. Interacting epidemics and gay men's health: A theory of syndemic production among urban gay men. In: Wolitski RJ, Stall R, Valdiserri RO, eds. Unequal opportunity: Health disparities affecting gay and bisexual men in the United States. New York: Oxford University Press, 2008:251-74.

[10] Burks DJ, Robbins R, Durtschi JP. American Indian gay, bisexual and two-spirit men: A rapid assessment of HIV/AIDS risk factors, barriers to prevention and culturally-sensitive intervention. *Cult Health Sex* 2011;13:283-98.

[11] Sznitman S, Vanable PA, Carey MP, Brown LK, Valois RF, Stanton BF, et al. Using culturally sensitive media messages to reduce HIV-associated sexual behavior in high-risk African American adolescents: Results from a randomized trial. *J. Adolesc. Health* 2011;49:244-51.

[12] Salomon EA, Mimiaga MJ, Husnik MJ, Welles SL, Manseau MW, Montenegro AB, et al. Depressive symptoms, utilization of mental health care, substance use and sexual risk among young men who have sex with men in EXPLORE: Implications for age-specific interventions. *AIDS Behav.* 2009;13:811-21.

[13] Lovejoy TI, Heckman TG, Sikkema KJ, Hansen NB, Kochman A, Suhr JA, et al. Patterns and correlates of sexual activity and condom use behavior in persons 50-plus years of age living with HIV/AIDS. *AIDS Behav.* 2008;12:943-56.

[14] Broaddus MR, Schmiege SJ, Bryan AD. An expanded model of the temporal stability of condom use intentions: Gender-specific predictors among high-risk adolescents. *Ann. Behav. Med.* 2011;42:99-110.

[15] Dworkin SL, Fullilove RE, Peacock D. Are HIV/AIDS prevention interventions for heterosexually active men in the United States gender-specific? *Am. J. Public Health* 2009;99:981-4.

[16] Aguilera S, Plascencia AV. Culturally appropriate HIV/AIDS and substance abuse prevention programs for urban Native youth. *J. Psychedelic Drugs* 2005;37:299-304.

[17] Sabato TM, Silverio AQ. A forgotten population: Addressing comprehensive HIV prevention needs among American Asians and Pacific Islanders. *J. Assoc. Nurs. AIDS Care* 2010;21:364-70.

[18] Sandfort TGM, Dodge B. '...And then there was the down low': Introduction to Black and Latino male bisexualities. *Arch. Sex Behav.* 2008;37:675-82.

[19] Silenzio VMB. Anthropological assessment for culturally appropriate interventions targeting men who have sex with men. *Am. J. Public Health*2003;93:867-71.

Social science aspects

In: Human Immunodeficiency Virus …
Editors: Hugh Klein and Joav Merrick

ISBN: 978-1-62081-293-8

Chapter I

Condom use measurement in adolescent HIV prevention research: Is briefer better?

Christopher D. Houck[1,*], Angela Stewart[2], Larry K. Brown[1] and the Project SHIELD Study Group

[1]Bradley/Hasbro Children's Research Center and the Warren Alpert Medical School at Brown University, Providence, Rhode Island, US

[2]Bradley Hospital, Providence, Rhode Island, US

Abstract

Self-report measures of condom use are frequently used to determine the efficacy of HIV prevention programs, however, little is known about which condom use formats yield the most reliable data. Our study was conducted to determine how often adolescents respond reliably across three formats of condom use (dichotomous, ordinal, and continuous) and whether participant characteristics are associated with inconsistency. Survey data were collected from 1,190 adolescents, 15-21 years, participating in a behavioral HIV-prevention trial. Approximately 40% were inconsistent in their reports of condom use. Participant characteristics were not associated with consistency in responding. We conclude that single items of condom use may suffice for some purposes, but more precise measurement may require multiple formats.

Introduction

Other than abstinence, correct and consistent condom use is the most effective method for preventing HIV/AIDS. Increasing condom use among adolescents is a target of many HIV

* Correspondence: Christopher D Houck, PhD, Bradley/Hasbro Children's Research Center, One Hoppin Street, Suite 204, Providence, RI 02903, United States. Telephone: 404-444-8539. Fax: 401-444-4645. Email: chouck@lifespan.org.

prevention interventions, and demonstrating the efficacy of these interventions often relies on establishing condom use behavior change. However, there is no "gold standard" for condom use measurement and all such measures are subject to threats to validity and reliability. A review of the literature identified more than 70 measures of condom use in studies that correlated condom use with sexual risk behavior [1]. Among the studies reviewed, the most common formats were ordinal frequency measures asking how often condoms were used (36%), dichotomous formats with yes/no questions about condom use (28%), and proportional measures calculated from the number of protected sexual occasions divided by the total number of sexual occasions (21%).

Little is known about which condom use measurement formats yield the most reliable and valid data among adolescents. One study found that although adolescent reports of sexual behaviors such as engaging in vaginal sex in the last three months (kappa = .72) and number of lifetime sexual partners (intraclass correlation (ICC) = .81) were moderately to highly consistent when test-retest reliability was measured over a two-week period, consistency regarding use of condoms during last sex (kappa = .62) and participant counts of unprotected vaginal sex acts in a three-month period (ICC = .44) were lower, suggesting that condom use measures may be more vulnerable to threats to reliability [2]. Another study found significant inconsistencies among college students in their responses on two measures of condom use [3]. Sixty-three percent of respondents indicated that using condoms 18-19 out of 20 times represented "always" using a condom; however, one or two unprotected sex acts represents significantly greater risk than zero. Similar results have been found among high-risk heterosexually active adults [4]. Together, these studies suggest that condom use measures are also subject to threats to validity.

Little is known about adolescent participant characteristics associated with unreliable reports on measures of condom use. Other literatures provide clues regarding patterns of unreliable responding. From the substance use literature, Farrell and colleagues [5] found that 33% of adolescents provided inconsistent responses between drug use measured dichotomously (yes/no) and continuously (days used in past month). Those who inconsistently responded reported higher rates of nearly half of the drugs measured than those who were consistent, suggesting that inconsistency in response may be associated with more risk behavior. From the adult sexual risk literature, discrepancies in reports of sexual risk behavior based on data collection method are common, such that the average magnitude of combined underreporting and overreporting discrepancies in unprotected sex was 54% when retrospective surveys were compared to a daily diary method [6]. Participants, however, tended to underreport with the retrospective measure relative to the daily diary measure, suggesting that responses may vary depending on the type of measure used to collect data. Gender and sexual orientation were related to accuracy of report, such that MSM were more accurate than heterosexual men or women.

Accurate condom use measurement has direct implications for preventing HIV and other STIs and for public health policies. However, researchers often face dilemmas deciding which condom use measures to use with adolescents. The apparent accuracy of partner-by-partner measures of condom use that yield proportion data may be appealing. However, the burden placed on participants, poor recall accuracy for those with many sexual occasions, and participant frustration that may result from being asked many similar questions may be undesirable. Single items that ask respondents to estimate the frequency of condom use may be appealing for their simplicity, yet researchers may be concerned about the accuracy of data collected by this format because of cognitive biases that may influence responses, such as emphasizing recent or salient events or poor estimating skills.

Little information is available regarding the reliability of different formats of condom use assessments with adolescents. Thus, the present study compared congruence of adolescent responses to three formats (dichotomous, ordinal, and continuous) to determine whether these formats yield similar or disparate data. These data are expected to help guide recommendations for researchers in selecting condom use measures for adolescents. This study also examines associations between unreliable responding and participant characteristics (e.g., younger age) to determine whether disparate responses to different condom use formats are associated with greater risk behavior or demographic characteristics of participants. We expected to find congruence for the majority of participants between ordinal and continuous measures, but less agreement between dichotomous assessment (i.e., condom use at last intercourse) and the other formats (e.g., proportion of condom use) because a single protected or unprotected sex act may not be representative of a pattern of sexual behavior. We anticipated no demographic associations with unreliability as there was no literature among adolescents to support such hypotheses, but expected that more sex risk behavior (e.g., having sex with someone the same day they met) and more general risk behavior (e.g., legal arrests) would be related to greater unreliability in responding since greater frequency of risky behaviors may make accurate recall more difficult [5,7,8].

Our study

Detailed study procedures for Project SHIELD, an HIV prevention program, are described elsewhere [9]. Data were collected as part of a multi-site, randomized trial of a brief HIV prevention intervention for adolescents ages 15 to 21 from three US cities (Providence, RI; Atlanta, GA; Miami, FL). Data for the present analyses were available from 1,190 adolescents. Adolescents were recruited for Project SHIELD from primary care clinics and through outreach activities, including posters, flyers, street outreach, and referrals from friends. Adolescents were privately screened to determine whether they were eligible for the study. The inclusion criterion was having engaged in at least one episode of unprotected vaginal or anal sex in the past 90 days. Exclusion criteria were being currently pregnant, attempting to become pregnant, having given birth in the last 90 days, or currently participating in another HIV prevention study. Adolescents were also excluded if they self-reported being HIV-positive, as the aim of the study was primary prevention.

Rhode Island Hospital, Miriam Hospital, University of Miami, and Emory University institutional review boards approved study procedures, and informed consent was obtained from all participants or their guardians. Adolescents completed baseline assessments via audio computer-assisted self-interview (ACASI) to ensure privacy. Assessments were conducted either individually or in a group format with research staff present to answer questions and ensure privacy. Calendars and scripted cues were provided to assist in recall of 90-day time periods. Participants were compensated $50 for their time and effort.

The questionnaire was largely derived from measures used in an HIV prevention trial for high-risk young adults, Project LIGHT, where they demonstrated adequate internal reliability and sensitivity to intervention impact [10]. On average, the ACASI took approximately 45 minutes to complete and assessed variables previously shown to be related to HIV risk, including engaging in sex with someone in the past 90 days whom the participant had met the same day, age at first sexual intercourse, a history of previous suicide attempt, and arrest histories [11-14]. Questions related to condom use appeared in the first third of the questionnaire, following a series of demographic questions. Urine assays were conducted for three sexually transmitted infections (STIs): gonorrhea, Chlamydia, and trichomoniasis.

Condom use was measured in three formats, in the following order: dichotomous, ordinal, and continuous. 1) For the dichotomous measure, participants were asked to consider their last episode of vaginal or anal sex and respond either "yes" or "no" to the question "The last time you had sex, did you or the other person use a condom?" 2) For the ordinal measure, participants were asked to respond to the question "In the last 90 days, how often did you use a condom when you had vaginal or anal sex?" with five options: "never," "less than half the time," "about half the time," "more than half the time," and "always." The dichotomous and ordinal measures were separated by three questions, on separate screens, related to substance use during sex and recent sexual activity. 3) Finally, for the continuous measure, the proportion of times a condom was used was calculated for each participant. Participants reported the number of partners with whom they had had vaginal or anal sex in the past 90 days. For up to three partners, participants reported the number of vaginal and anal intercourse acts for each partner, followed by the number of times condoms were used during those acts, yielding a proportion of protected sex acts. These partner-specific questions, used to generate a continuous measure of condom use, immediately followed the ordinal assessment.

Data analysis was approached by comparing the responses of the three condom use assessment formats completed by all participants. First, rates of endorsement were compared with the three forms of measurement. The mean proportion of condom use (continuous measurement) was calculated for each response option for the ordinal item "In the last 90 days, how often did you use a condom when you had vaginal or anal sex?" (i.e., "never," "less than half the time," "about half the time," "more than half the time," and "always"; see Table 1, Column A). Similarly, the percentage who reported "yes" to having used a condom at last sex (dichotomous measurement) for each ordinal response option was calculated (see Table 1, Column B).

Next, each participant was coded as a "reliable" or "unreliable" reporter based on the match between his/her responses on the continuous and the ordinal measures. Participants were deemed reliable if the proportion of condom use (p) calculated from their partner-specific reports matched the ordinal grouping that they selected using the following ranges: $p = 100\%$ and "always"; $100\% > p \geq 60\%$ and "more than half the time"; $60\% > p \geq 40\%$ and "about half the time"; $40\% > p > 0\%$ and "less than half the time"; or $p = 0\%$ and "never." Then, Pearson Chi-square and t-test analyses were conducted to assess for differences on demographic and behavioral variables between participants who were reliable and those who were not.

Our findings

The sample was 56% female, with an average age of 18.8 years. The racial/ethnic composition of the sample was representative of the communities where the study was conducted. Fifty-two percent of the sample identified as Black or African American, 23% as Hispanic, 20% as White, and 5% as "Other." Ninety-two percent of the sample identified as heterosexual, 5% as bisexual, 3% as undecided, and 1% as homosexual.

Twenty percent reported currently living with a spouse or partner. Approximately 49% of the sample had completed 11th grade or less at the time of the study, 27% had completed the twelfth grade or obtained a GED, and 24% had completed some college or technical school education. Regarding socioeconomic status, 17% indicated that they were currently receiving public assistance.

The sample reported high rates of risk behavior. The mean proportion of condom use in the last 90 days for the total sample was .38. The percentage of participants who used a condom at last intercourse was also 38%. The average number of sex partners was 2.1 (SD = 2.4), with 6.8% reporting more than three partners in the past 90 days. The mean age at sexual debut was 14.5 years (SD = 2.5). Approximately 14% tested positive for an STI on urine screen, and 13.5% indicated that they had had sex in the last 90 days with a partner the same day that they had met him/her. Nineteen percent reported that they had tried to kill themselves at some time during their lifetime, and 35% said that they had been arrested on at least one previous occasion.

Comparing the continuous and dichotomous assessments, the proportion of condom use in the past 90 days was significantly higher among those who used a condom the last time they had sex than among those who did not (0.70 vs. 0.23; $t(1{,}186\ df) = -25.5$, $p < .001$). Table 1 shows the relationship between participant responses to the ordinal descriptors and their responses on the continuous and dichotomous formats. Both indicate linear patterns consistent with the ordinal descriptors.

Sixty-one percent of participants reliably responded to the ordinal and continuous assessments for the past 90 days. When participants were unreliable, they more often indicated greater condom use on the ordinal item than they endorsed on questions generating the proportion of condom use (see Table 1).

Table 1. Rates of condom use by response on a brief, ordinal condom use measure

Categories of condom use	n	A Continuous Mean(SD)	B Dichoto-mous	Consistent between continuous and ordinal measures	Ordinal response greater than continuous measure	Ordinal response less than continuous measure
Never	307	.3 (.13)	3%	85%	NA	15%
Less than half the time	269	.26 (.26)	19%	51%	25%	24%
About half the time	206	.44 (.27)	37%	35%	38%	27%
More than half the time	280	.70 (.27)	66%	58%	26%	15%
Always	128	.91 (.23)	98%	76%	24%	NA

Bivariate analyses were conducted to examine whether demographic or behavioral differences existed between participants who responded reliably and those who did not. Results suggest that unreliable responders were younger ($t(928) = 2.68$, $p = .007$), had fewer instances of unprotected sex ($t(1,159) = 5.39$, $p < .001$), were more likely to be African American (χ^2 (2) = 18.50, $p < .001$), and were more likely to have an STI on the urine test (χ^2 (1) = 6.07, $p = .014$). No significant differences emerged related to gender, sexual orientation, number of sexual partners, age at sexual debut, proportion of sex acts with a condom in the last 90 days, sex with someone met the same day, a history of suicide attempt, or a history of legal arrest.

Youth who never used condoms formed the largest group of consistent responders. With this in mind, we considered that this large group of reliable, but particularly risky, adolescents may have strongly influenced the bivariate differences noted above. Because of this potential confounding between consistency and sexual risk (i.e., never using condoms), analyses comparing reliable and unreliable responders on demographic and behavioral variables were conducted again omitting adolescents who endorsed never using condoms. After removing this group, no significant differences remained between reliable and unreliable reporters on age, race, number of unprotected sex acts, or STI results.

Discussion

These data suggest that brief and detailed assessments of condom use in the last 90 days yield consistent responses in approximately 60% of cases, indicating that the majority of adolescents interpret these assessment methods similarly and respond reliably. At a group level, reports of condom use at last sex also corresponded to continuous and ordinal formats. However, 40% of youth were inconsistent in their reporting, which may represent a serious concern for those conducting research or program evaluations.

Rates of reliable responding were highest at the extremes of condom use (“always” and “never”). It would appear that these patterns of use are easiest for adolescents to quantify and lead to the highest rates of reliability. However, some inconsistency emerged even in the extreme ends of the ordinal variable (“always” and “never”). Similar to adults [3], adolescents’ interpretation of “always” may include less than 100% of the time and their definition of “never” may include more than 0%. More detail in defining these categories for teens, such as providing corresponding percentages, may be useful in future assessments.

Inconsistency in responding occurred most frequently among adolescents reporting occasional condom use. In fact, the two least reliable groups were those endorsing “less than half the time” and “about half the time.” These individuals are often the focus of intervention programs aimed at encouraging the consistent use of condoms among those willing to use them, but doing so sporadically. Research suggests that occasional condom users are at high risk for HIV [15] and therefore should be targeted for intervention. However, accurate condom use measurement among this “occasional” group may be a significant barrier to quantifying behavior change. Multiple measures may be necessary with this population.

When participants were unreliable, they tended to estimate more condom use on the ordinal format than they did on the continuous one. While it is not possible to establish which is the more accurate response, the tendency for adolescents to estimate greater condom use when responding to frequency measures is important when drawing conclusions based on data derived from single ordinal items. Thus, studies using ordinal condom measurement should be aware of possible response biases that underestimate risk behavior when interpreting findings.

There are limitations to this study. Since objective assessment of condom use in the sample is unavailable, none of these measures can be established as a "gold standard." However, computer-assisted survey instruments, like those used in this study, have been shown minimize some of the limitations associated with self-reports of private information and to increase accuracy [6, 16]. Also, since all participants were recruited because they had recent unprotected sex, this sample was high risk; how lower-risk adolescents might interpret these items is unknown. However, previous work with adults has suggested that those who report more frequent sexual behavior on (presumably more accurate) daily diaries are less consistent in retrospective reports than those with fewer behaviors [6]. Therefore, one might conclude that less risky youth might be more reliable reporters.

Despite recruiting adolescents who reported a recent episode of unprotected sex, some participants reported consistent condom use during the period of time assessed. Oftentimes, the initial eligibility screening (determining whether adolescents had unprotected sex in the last 90 days) was separated in time from the computer assessment due to arranging appointments for informed consent and assessment procedures. Therefore, an eligible adolescent's last episode of unprotected sex may have fallen outside the window of the last 90 days by the time of the computer assessment. In addition, adolescents may have misunderstood or misled staff during the eligibility screen. However, this may also be to the benefit of the current study, as it provided at least some representation of youth who were consistently using condoms.

Minority participants comprised a greater percentage of the sample than is representative of the United States as a whole. While the racial/ethnic composition was representative of the communities in which the study took place and represents three U.S. cities, these findings may not be generalizable to other populations. For example, African-American youth often report earlier sexual debut than other racial/ethnic groups [17]; the impact of how more sexual experience might influence reliability in reporting is unknown. Finally, the order in which these formats were presented may have influenced the response; this study was not designed to assess the impact of the order in which these items were administered. For example, had the partner-by-partner (i.e., continuous) assessment been presented first, rather than last, participants may have been primed to more carefully consider their sexual experiences over the past three months and respond more consistently to the broader, ordinal assessment item.

Social science implications

These findings have significant implications for studies of adolescent risk behavior, as they provide important information regarding the reliability of adolescent reports of condom use. Since there was general agreement across formats, assessment of condom use at last sex may be sufficient for some purposes. Otherwise, adolescents, while often reliable, tended to report more condom use on brief, ordinal measures than detailed, continuous ones, thus the measure of condom use should be taken into account when interpreting research findings. Therefore, precise assessment of changes in condom use rates, the goal of many HIV prevention studies, may require multiple measures.

A large percentage of adolescents (40%) were inconsistent in reporting condom use across different formats, and it was difficult to discern factors associated with inconsistency. This confirms problematic responding that has been similarly observed with adults, where the rate of disagreement in number of unprotected sex acts by adult reports on daily diaries compared with 3-month retrospective surveys averaged 54% [6]. Given that all of the accounts of unprotected sex in the current study were retrospective, it suggests that formatting of the items may influence how adolescents respond. Among adults, McAuliffe and colleagues [6] have found that partner-by-partner assessment techniques have been found to be more reliable than aggregate assessment strategies (asking for total numbers of behaviors summed across partners). While the current study does not allow for conclusions as to which assessment methods were most accurate, researchers may wish to incorporate some partner-by-partner assessment with adolescent samples.

At the same time, the disadvantages of brief methods of condom use assessment must be weighed against the disadvantages of more comprehensive strategies. As noted elsewhere [6], the use of more intensive strategies of collecting accurate data should not lead participants to alter their responses. Among the methods studied here, the potential exists for adolescents to become inattentive or impatient with partner-by-partner questions that involve detailed follow-up questions. As a result, they may reduce the number of partners they endorse or misrepresent their engagement in sexual activity altogether to shorten the time required of the survey. This especially may be a concern in studies with repeated follow-ups, in which adolescents over the duration of the study may grow savvy to the consequences of endorsing sexual activity and the benefits of denying sexual activity. Studies examining patterns of responding over time are needed to answer these important questions.

Initial results suggested that African-American youth and adolescents with a STI-positive urine assay were more likely to be unreliable. Also, inconsistent responders reported fewer unprotected sex acts in the last 90 days. As mentioned, the most inconsistent response options were in the middle of the ordinal scale (i.e., using condoms some, but not all of the time), thus when compared to peers who consistently reported never using condoms, they had fewer unprotected acts. However, after the removal of those who reported "never" using condoms (who also tended to be consistent in their reporting) these differences no longer existed, suggesting that the riskiest youth in the sample were influencing these effects. By eliminating the variability in STIs and unprotected sex associated with this subgroup, these factors were no longer associated with inconsistent responding.

Similarly, analyses of the whole sample suggested that younger participants were less consistent in reporting than older ones, though this difference did not persist when the riskiest adolescents were removed from the analysis. Again, inattentiveness may be associated with this finding. Alternatively, younger adolescents may have been reluctant to acknowledge socially stigmatized behavior and thus underreported lack of condom use when asked repeatedly. These influences of age on reporting cannot be assessed in the present study, but should be investigated further.

The social science evidence provided in the current study informs the field regarding strategies for assessing sexual risk behavior and populations for whom special attention might be paid when assessing condom use and looking for change. Adolescents and young adults at the extremes of the behavior, either never using condoms or always using them, appear to be consistent in their reports, and can likely be accurately assessed with either detailed or brief measurement. However, when assessing those in the middle, often of interest in prevention studies, more targeted assessment strategies may be needed.

Acknowledgments

Project SHIELD Study Group Principal Investigators: Larry Brown, MD, Rhode Island Hospital, Providence, RI; Ralph DiClemente, PhD, Emory University, Atlanta, GA; M Isabel Fernandez, PhD, University of Miami, Miami, FL, Timothy Flanigan, MD, Miriam Hospital, Providence, RI; Deborah Haller, PhD, Virginia Commonwealth University, Richmond, VA; Lori Leonard, ScD, University of Texas, Houston Health Science Center, Houston, TX; Lydia O'Donnell, EdD, Education Development Center, Inc., Newton, MA; William E Schlenger, PhD, Research Triangle Institute, Research Triangle Park, NC; Barbara Silver, PhD, Substance Abuse and Mental Health Services Administration, Rockville, MD. Site Investigators: Richard Crosby, PhD, Emory University, Atlanta, GA; Caryl Gay, PhD, University of Miami, Miami, FL; Janet Knisely, PhD, Virginia Commonwealth University, Richmond, VA; Celia Lescano, PhD, Rhode Island Hospital, Providence, RI; Kevin Lourie, PhD, Rhode Island Hospital, Providence, RI; Louise Masse, PhD, University of Texas, Houston Health Science Center, Houston, TX; Janet O'Connell, MPH, Miriam Hospital, Providence, RI; David Pugatch, MD, Miriam Hospital, Providence, RI; Eve Rose, PhD, Emory University, Atlanta, GA; Ann Stueve, PhD, Columbia School of Public Health, New York, NY; Leah Varga, MA, University of Miami, Miami, FL; Sue Vargo, PhD, Education Development Center, Inc., Newton, MA; Gina Wingood, ScD, MPH, Emory University, Atlanta, GA. Coordinating Center Investigators, Research Triangle Institute, Research Triangle Park, NC: Jamia L Bacharach, JD, Sylvia Cohn, Courtney Johnson, PhD, Jacquelyn R Murphy, BSc, Allison Rose, PhD and Scott Royal, PhD, MPH. Consumer Representatives: Christian Aldridge, Beri Hull and Sean Scott. This research was supported by SAMHSA grant U10 SMS2073 to the cooperating sites: Rhode Island Hospital, Miriam Hospital, Emory University, and University of Miami, and by the Lifespan/Brown/Tufts Center for AIDS Research.

References

[1] Noar SM, Cole C, Carlyle K. Condom use measurement in 56 studies of sexual risk behavior: Review and recommendations. *Arch. Sex Behav.* 2006;35:327-45.

[2] Vanable PA, Carey MP, Brown JL, DiClemente RJ, Salazar LF, Brown LK, Romer D, et al. Test-retest reliability of self-reported HIV/STD-related measures among African-American adolescents in four U.S. cities. *J. Adolesc. Health* 2009;44:214-21.

[3] Cecil H, Zimet GD. Meanings assigned by undergraduates to frequency statements of condom use. *Arch. Sex Behav.* 1998;27:493-505.

[4] White SL, Redding CA, Morokoff PJ, Meier KS, Rossi JS, Gazabon SA, et al. Utility of a 5-point Likert condom frequency scale in at risk sexually active adults. *Ann. Behav. Med.* 2000;22(Suppl):S075.

[5] Farrell AD, Danish SJ, Howard CW. Evaluation of data screening methods in surveys of adolescent drug use. *Psychol. Assess* 1991; 3:295-8.

[6] McAuliffe TL, DiFranceisco W, Reed BR. Effects of question format and collection mode on the accuracy of retrospective surveys of health risk behavior: A comparison with daily sexual activity diaries. *Health Psychol.* 2007;26:60-7.

[7] Brener ND, Billy JO, Grady WR. Assessment of factors affecting the validity of self-reported health-risk behavior among adolescents: Evidence from the scientific literature. *J. Adolesc. Health* 2003; 33:436-57.

[8] Catania JA, Gibson DR, Chitwood DD, Coates TJ. Methodological problems in AIDS behavioral research: Influences on measurement error and participation bias in studies of sexual behavior. *Psychol. Bull* 1990; 108:339-62.

[9] Brown LK, DiClemente R, Crosby R, Fernandez MI, Pugatch D, Cohn S, Lescano C, Royal S, Murphy JR, Silver B, Schlenger WE. Condom use among high-risk adolescents: Anticipation of partner disapproval and less pleasure associated with not using condoms. *Public Health Rep.* 2008; 123:601-7.

[10] NIMH Multisite HIV Prevention Trial Group. The NIMH multisite HIV prevention trial: Reducing HIV sexual risk behavior. *Science* 1999; 280:1889-94.

[11] Crosby R, DiClemente RJ, Wingood G, Salazar LF, Rose E, Levine D, et al. Correlates of condom failure among adolescent males: An exploratory study. *Prev. Med.* 2005;41:873-6.

[12] O'Donnell L, O'Donnell CR, Stueve, A. Early sexual initiation and subsequent sex-related risks among urban minority youth: The Reach for Health study. *Fam. Plann Perspect* 2001;33:268-75.

[13] Houck CD, Hadley W, Lescano CM, Pugatch D, Brown LK, Project SHIELD Study Group. Suicide attempt and sexual risk behavior: Relationship among adolescents. *Arch. Suicide Res.* 2008;12:39-49.

[14] Tolou-Shams M, Brown LK, Gordon G, Fernandez MI. Arrest history as an indicator of adolescent/young adult substance abuse and HIV risk. *Drug Alcohol Depend.* 2007; 88:87-90.

[15] Weir SS, Roddy RE, Zekeng L, Ryan KA. Association between condom use and HIV infection: A randomised study of self reported condom use measures. *J. Epidemiol. Commun. Health* 1999;53:417-22.

[16] Romer D, Hornik RC, Stanton B, Black M, Li X, Ricardo I, Feigelman S. "Talking" computers: A private and reliable method to conduct interviews on sensitive topics with children. *J. Sex Res.* 1997;34:3-9.

[17] Cavazos-Rehg PA, Krauss MJ, Spitznagel EL, Schootman M, Bucholz KK, Peipert JF, Sanders-Thompson V, Cottler LB, Bierut LJ. Age of sexual debut among US adolescents. *Contraception* 2009;80:158-62.

In: Human Immunodeficiency Virus …
Editors: Hugh Klein and Joav Merrick

ISBN: 978-1-62081-293-8

Chapter II

Internet advice on disclosure of HIV status to sexual partners in an era of criminalization

Bronwen Lichtenstein*
Department of Criminal Justice, University of Alabama,
Tuscaloosa, Alabama, US

Abstract

HIV-specific statutes are increasingly popular in the United States and often impose harsh penalties for failure to disclose an HIV diagnosis to sexual partners. The purpose of this study was to examine HIV-related websites for information about non-disclosure as a crime and the relevance of this advice for US audiences. Internet searches were conducted for HIV-related websites with advice on disclosure to sexual partners. Once identified, these sites were analyzed for content, quality, and type of approach to disclosure and the law. Each site was given a page ranking (P. Score) according to Google's priority listing algorithm, and a value ranking (V. Score) for textual content and quality of advice. Internet advice on disclosure and the law was highly variable. With few exceptions, highly ranked US sites offered less advice than sites in Britain, Canada and Australia. All US sites followed the law by placing the onus of responsibility for disclosure on the HIV-infected individual, but few offered advice on how to disclose or how to obtain proof of disclosure in order to avoid prosecution. None addressed the special risks of African Americans who are most likely to be prosecuted for non-disclosure. It is concluded that HIV advice websites should offer strategies on how to disclose to sexual partners and to document proof in case of prosecution.

* Correspondence: Bronwen Lichtenstein, PhD, Department of Criminal Justice. 430 Farrah Hall, University of Alabama, Tuscaloosa, AL 35487-0320 United States. Phone (205) 348 7782; Fax: (205) 348 7178; Email: blichten@ua.edu.

Introduction

HIV-specific statutes are increasingly popular in the United States and often impose harsh penalties for failure to disclose an HIV diagnosis to sexual partners [1]. General criminal law is also used to prosecute HIV-related acts involving non-disclosure [1]. The precursors to criminalizing HIV non-disclosure arose from moral panics of the 1980s when epidemiologists at the Centers for Disease Control and Prevention (CDC) coined the term "the four H's" to describe homosexuals, heroin users, hookers, and Haitians as risk groups for HIV/AIDS [2]. Since marginalized people were viewed as disease bearers from the outset, it is perhaps inevitable that HIV-related behavior was criminalized in the U.S. and that non-disclosure to sexual partners became the lynchpin of efforts to include HIV-specific statutes in the canon of criminal law.

The legal requirements for disclosure were embedded in the Ryan White Care Act of 1990, in which states had to agree to prosecute cases of "intentional" HIV exposure in order to receive federal funding for HIV care [3].

The 1990s thus became a watershed decade for HIV-specific laws in which non-disclosure was considered to be a criminal act, particularly if an "innocent" partner became infected heterosexually [3,4]. The increase in criminalization for HIV-related cases in the U.S. is consistent with trends in other Western countries [5].

However, the U.S. has led the way with more prosecutions of HIV-related acts involving non-disclosure or threats to public safety than anywhere else in the world [6].

Evolving law on criminal non-disclosure

US case law on HIV-related crime has evolved over the past 30 years. In the 1980s, non-disclosure of positive HIV serostatus could be prosecuted under existing public health statutes that allowed states to charge people who willfully or knowingly exposed someone to infectious diseases that were a threat to public health. This provision included prosecutions for sexually transmitted infections (STIs) such as syphilis and gonorrhea [7]. However, the misdemeanors that could be imposed for breaching public health laws were too lenient for many lawmakers who sought harsher penalties for HIV exposure than public health statutes would allow [8]. By 1990, 23 states had enacted HIV-specific laws that were designed to control disease and punish wrongdoers [1]. A decade later, HIV-specific laws had been enacted in 34 states, and sexual and even non-sexual acts such as spitting, biting, or throwing tainted blood, were being prosecuted under general criminal law [1]. In some cases, non-disclosure was being prosecuted even if the accused was unaware of being HIV-infected [10].

General criminal law is widely used to prosecute non-disclosure and non-sexual acts that are perceived to be risky for police officers and other first responders. HIV-infected people have been charged with criminal exposure, aggravated or felonious assault/assault with a deadly weapon, sexual battery, rape, reckless endangerment and murder regardless of whether or not HIV transmission or even sexual activity took place. Once convicted, HIV-infected people often receive enhanced penalties because of the perceived seriousness of their crimes [1,11]. HIV was criminalized further in the wake of 9/11 when prosecutorial desire to impose penalties for HIV-related behavior received a boost from new laws to combat terrorism. This expansion of law meant that threatening to infect someone with HIV was considered a "terroristic threat" and, in one notable case, was prosecuted as a case of bioterrorism [12].

The upward trend in HIV-related arrests and prosecutions is evident in statistical reports. By 2010, a total of 375 arrests and prosecutions – a low estimate – were documented in the United States [1,11]. Almost 30 percent of these cases (n=109) were prosecuted between 2008 and 2011 alone, an increase that is variously attributed to media sensationalism, public outrage, harsher sentencing, and even having to register as a sex offender for life [1,13,14]. Public health campaigns that were once popular in promoting shared responsibility by both partners to establish sexual histories, discuss safer sex, and use condoms failed to curtail this trend, perhaps because of the multiplying effects of harsher social attitudes toward sexual crimes, epidemiologic trends in race-gender disparities in HIV/AIDS, and the highly-charged contexts in which most prosecutions occurred.

Public health models for HIV prevention

In the mid-1980s, public health approaches to HIV prevention focused on a particular message: People should inquire about the sexual history of potential partners before having sex [15]. This approach to safer sex, termed "the mutual (shared) responsibility" model, recommended seeking information about sexual orientation, drug use, frequency of sexual activity, and STI history as a means of assessing HIV risk [16]. The approach was the model of choice for HIV prevention, primarily because of the public health sector's reluctance to place the burden of responsibility solely on HIV-infected people who were already heavily stigmatized as putative AIDS vectors [17]. The goals of the campaign were to promote co-equal information sharing, full disclosure of HIV status, and mutual responsibility for initiating condom use. The model assumed that sexual actors would be both self-empowered and self-motivated to engage in safer sex. However, a campaign that was designed primarily for HIV seropositive or at-risk men in the gay community was not always relevant to other actors, especially African Americans and women. Wingood and DiClemente [18] reported that African American women were ill served by public health directives to initiate safer sex with sexual partners. Such women were often accused of sexual cheating and undermining male authority, and, rather than being self-empowered, sometimes faced threats of violence and abandonment as a result of attempts to negotiate condom use.

By the late 1980s, the individual (personal) responsibility model for HIV disclosure, also known as the altruism or "responsibility for the other" approach [19] had gained influence among policymakers [17]. According to Bayer [20], many HIV prevention specialists opposed this approach because they believed it would intensify HIV stigma for highly vulnerable groups in society. Nevertheless, ethics concerns over the special responsibilities of HIV-infected persons in a deadly epidemic, and the potential for HIV transmission in the absence of disclosure, provided the impetus for widespread acceptance of the personal responsibility approach to HIV prevention [20]. The model posited that HIV-infected people must disclose their seropositive status prior to sexual activity, and also to assume responsibility for both disclosure and safer sex. Mutual exchange of information between sexual partners, and shared responsibility for safer sex were no longer a public health priority. The CDC formalized the individual responsibility model in a report titled "Advancing HIV prevention: New strategies for a changing epidemic – United States 2003" [17]. The link between the individualistic approach to HIV prevention and legal enforcement of this approach was underwritten in expectations of "contractual responsibility," in which recipients of HIV care were fully responsible for HIV disclosure [19]. As noted, this change in public health policy meant that U.S. citizens who received public HIV care could be prosecuted if they failed to disclose their HIV seropositive status to sexual partners [3].

The law versus medicine

The law enforcement approach to HIV non-disclosure to sexual partners is at odds with recent medical advances in HIV care. First, the advent of antiretroviral medicines (ARVs) meant that HIV-infected people were able to lead longer and healthier lives [21] in which the chances of HIV transmission were greatly reduced when ARVs were taken as prescribed [22]. On the basis of these advances, the CDC promoted routine HIV testing in the belief that early diagnosis and treatment would save lives and prevent transmission to sexual partners [23]. This recommendation took account of the life-saving benefits of the new HIV drugs, but did not reduce the burden of disclosure for HIV-infected people. If anything, the policy meant that people who heeded the CDC's recommendation for early testing and were then diagnosed with HIV suddenly faced the prospect of legally circumscribed sexual activity on a permanent basis. Second, rather than recognize the changing medical landscape for HIV transmission, lawmakers increased their efforts to impose stiff penalties on HIV-infected people who were assumed to place others at risk by failing to disclose their HIV status.

What accounts for this divergence between medicine and the law? Critics have charged that stigma rather than medical evidence drove the zeal to criminalize non-disclosure, particularly in cases involving heterosexuals [4]. As a case in point, HIV is often compared to infectious diseases such as Hepatitis B or C, also acquired through injection drug use or unprotected sex. After HIV emerged as a public health threat in the 1980s, these less sensationalized conditions did not attract the same stigma despite high rates of morbidity and even mortality [24,25]. Unlike HIV, exposure to Hepatitis B and C is rarely prosecuted under public health statutes and even more rarely under general criminal law [26].

Broad social trends and epidemiologic changes can help to explain recent trends in criminalization. Poverty [27], drug use [27], minority ethnic status [28], and mental illness [29] are all indicators of HIV risk in the United States. African Americans are 10 times more likely than Whites to acquire HIV/AIDS, a disparity that has widened over time [28]. Furthermore, today's criminal cases are driven mostly by heterosexual rather than same-sex acts, particularly if they involve Black men [4,29,30,31]. This racial patterning suggests that social factors and, perhaps, racial stereotyping are at work in re-stigmatizing HIV. The hardening public attitudes toward acts that classify as sexual offenses [32] have also contributed to harsher attitudes toward HIV non-disclosure. These attitudes were driven, in part, by media sensationalism over sex crimes [33], so that people who fail to disclose an HIV-positive diagnosis were likely to be perceived as sexual predators, especially if they were male [11]. History has shown that public attitudes toward issues of race/ethnicity, gender, and sexuality are particularly potent when it comes to the law [34].

Criminalization leads to fear of being tested for HIV [35,36], and to erroneous beliefs that non-disclosure of seropositive HIV status to sexual partners is driving the epidemic, despite evidence that the lack of HIV testing and treatment is a greater problem [37]. The success of HIV criminalization as an HIV prevention tool is certainly in question; new HIV cases in the U.S. have remained stubbornly high, at around 56,000 annually over the past decade [38]. Persson and Newman [4] wrote that the law enforcement approach to HIV non-disclosure is counterproductive, and involves blame motifs involving perpetrators and victims [4] "in a revival and reframing of the old familiar discourse of 'innocent victims' and 'guilty others' so prevalent in early news reporting" (p. 633). This polarization is at the heart of high-profile cases in which HIV-infected men such as Nushawn Williams, an African American man who infected mostly White women, have been prosecuted for non-disclosure. Scholars argue that the refocus on individual responsibility represents a victim-perpetrator antagonism which, in the words of Galletly and Pinkerton [39]: "Reinforces the 'them versus us' dichotomy that is central to prevailing theories of stigma" (p. 457). Indeed, fears over this type of stigmatization were the original impetus for formulating the mutual responsibility model when moral panics over HIV were at their peak in the 1980s. The transition to the individual responsibility model signals a maturing epidemic, as well as a law and order approach to infection control after HIV was associated with sexual crime and, not incoincidentally, communities of color.

The disclosure dilemma

Legal enforcement of HIV-positive status ignores the difficulties of disclosing to sexual partners. Serovich and Mosack [40] reported that perhaps 50% of HIV-infected people do not disclose to sexual partners for fear of being rejected, abandoned, or even assaulted. The criminalization of non-disclosure presents a new wrinkle among HIV-infected people: Risk rejection or even violence if you disclose and prosecution if you do not. Being liable for prosecution begins even before deciding whether or not to disclose to sexual partners. Few people are aware that HIV-specific statutes override confidentiality laws when someone is charged with an HIV-related crime and that medical records can be subpoenaed as evidence for the prosecution [41]. In other words, an HIV-positive diagnosis can be used against the accused in a court of law.

Most HIV-infected people are counseled about their rights and responsibilities at the time of diagnosis, including information about legal requirements for disclosure to sexual partners. In the Internet age, HIV-infected people are also likely to consult relevant websites on how to disclose to sexual partners, especially if they fear rejection, seek anonymity, or wish to be protected from legal jeopardy. The purpose of the present study was to examine the relevance of advice on HIV disclosure and the law for Internet users in the United States. The specific goals were to: 1) Identify websites that offer information on HIV disclosure and the law, 2) Identify the intended audience for U.S. websites, 3) Conduct a content analysis on quality of the advice, 4) Compare the search engine rankings with the quality of advice, and 5) Describe the approaches to such advice according to the Mutual Responsibility and Individual Responsibility models as described above.

The study

Ethics approval was obtained from the Institutional Review Board at the University of Alabama, which was followed by multiple Google searches using search terms such as "HIV disclosure," "Telling/Partner/HIV," and "How do I disclose HIV?" The searches were conducted on four different computers at home, work, and a computer laboratory in order to circumvent a process known as personalization, the method by which Google uses personal search histories and a page-rank algorithm to filter results [42]. This reiterative search produced more than 300 pages of results, mostly news items, legal documents, or scientific articles (they were discarded) as well as duplicated results for HIV-related websites. All relevant items were counted only once in the final tally. In the second stage of the research, a Priority Score (P. Score) was assigned to the remaining 113 items on HIV disclosure, that is, the page ranking assigned by the search engine itself. The most-highly ranked item was assigned a score of 1 ("highest accessibility") with other items ranked sequentially, ending with the 113th item on the list ("lowest accessibility").

The content analysis consisted of a detailed review of relevant websites for information on HIV disclosure and the law. Only 50 (44%) of the 113 websites on HIV disclosure had information or advice about disclosure and the law. A value ranking (V. Score) was assigned to these sites, as calculated from the amount of text and quality of advice. The amount and quality of information were closely related. This content was then ranked from 1 to 5, with the least helpful (one to two sentences) receiving a score of 1, moderately helpful (several paragraphs to one page) receiving scores of 2 and 3 respectively, and very helpful (multiple pages with links) receiving a score of 4. Only one website received the top score of 5 because it was entirely dedicated to HIV disclosure and the law.

Once the ranking was complete, the author identified sites that offered peer-to-peer advice (informal), doctor-patient or institutional-legal advice (formal), or some other type of approach to disclosure and the law. The research also assessed whether or not each website addressed disclosure according to evolving legal standards for public health policy and the law. Then, the study examined the type of approach ("shared responsibility" versus "individual responsibility") to see if the advice was tailored to client advocacy (the shared responsibility model), the law (the individual responsibility model), or some other approach. Finally, the target audience for each website was identified to determine if the advice was generic or crafted for a particular demographic or community.

Results

The results are organized into four sub-sections according to the specific research questions for the study. The first section describes the priority rankings that were generated by the search engine, and the relevance of these results for U.S. Internet users. This section is followed by an assessment of the quality of the advice on the most highly ranked sites, and approach to advice on HIV disclosure and the law. The third section analyzes the usefulness of advice on the top 10 ranked websites for US Internet users.

Table 1. HIV sites citing legal reasons for disclosure by Priority and Value Scores (N=21)

P. Score[1] Website	Audience	Tag line	V. Score[2]	Location
1. *AIDSmeds.com*	HIV+	To tell or not to tell	2	US
2. *Thewellproject.org*	HIV+ women	Hiv and disclosure	2	US
3. *Thebody.com*	HIV+	Should you disclose ... ?	4	US
4. *Webmd.com*	General	Telling others	1	US
5. *Mdjunction.com*	General	To tell or not to tell	2	US
6. *IPPF.org*	Youth	Some countries have laws	3	UK
9. *Gmfa.org.uk*	HIV+ men	Sexual transmission and law	4	UK
10. *Catie.ca*	HIV+	HIV, disclosure and the law	3	Canada
11. *Aidslex.org (law)*	HIV+	Disclosing your HIV status	5	Australia
12. *Friendsofaids.org*	HIV+	Ready to disclose?	1	US
13.*Positivewomensnetwork*	HIV+ women	Sex, HIV, and the law	3	Canada
14. Methedoctor.com	General	Some things to consider ...	2	Indonesia
20. Poz.com	HIV+	Daring to disclose	2	US
24. Pozitude.co.uk	HIV+	HIV, sex and the law	4	UK
26. Ehow.com	General	HIV disclosure laws	4	US, UK
30. Doh.state.fl.us	HIV+	Why is disclosure important?	3	US
39.Positivelypositive.ca	HIV+ men	Why is disclosure important?	3	Canada
40. Wdxcyber.com	Women	Relationships and HIV	1	US
41. HIVsa.org.au	HIV+	Know your rights!	3	Australia
47. AIDSlondon.com	HIV+	Disclosure	4	UK
50. Avert.org	HIV-related	Criminal transmission	4	UK

1. Numbers for the P. Score reflect the Internet rankings and are not in consecutive order.
2. Scores: One to two sentences =1; One or two short paragraphs =2; Half to one page=3; Multi-page or link=4; Entire report=5.

Finally, the question of: "whose responsibility?" is discussed in relation to website advice on disclosing to sexual partners within the framework of U.S. law.

Priority rankings

Only 44% of websites with advice on HIV disclosure provided information about the legal aspects of disclosing to sexual partners. Moreover, while 13 (65%) of the top 20 sites, as ranked by Google, addressed disclosure and the law – a reasonable showing - the percentage declined steadily thereafter. Table 1 presents a list of 21 U.S. and international sites that offered information on disclosure and the law (space limitations preclude listing all results in this category). These highly placed sites stood a reasonable chance of being read because they appeared in the top half of the rankings. Since the top five of these websites originated in the United States, the legal advice was relevant contextually to U.S. users. However, sites in the United Kingdom, Canada, and Australia ranked higher overall and were slightly more numerous as well. Compared to no-frills advice in four of the top U.S. websites, these foreign sites had detailed, friendly advice and even referrals to legal advisors if needed.

The top ranked U.S. websites offered multiple pages in the form of homepage, sections, videos, and links to other sites. Advertisements appeared for treatments and services within the site or on the page of Google results. The highest ranking (1/113) went to AIDSmeds.com, a New York-based advocacy network for people seeking advice on HIV treatment and clinical trials. The site was visually appealing, highly interactive, had news about HIV drugs and clinical trials, and provided ready access to affiliated sites for further information. Unlike other top ranked sites, AIDSmeds.com offered advice on disclosure and the law, which referred users to government services (e.g., "The Department of Public Health in your state is a good source of information about what the legal procedure is in your state and how it might apply to you"). Photographs, video clips, and graphics on the homepage suggested that the website catered to a cross-section of the HIV-infected community, although White men were typically depicted on the main page and links. The superior ranking of this site reflected its popularity in providing information on treatment advances and new developments in clinical care and, of course, advertising links to expensive, name brand HIV drugs. The site offered a link to RealHealth, a health website for African Americans, but the absence of an exclusive or even primary focus on HIV/AIDS on RealHealth suggests that the site lacked relevance for HIV-infected African Americans seeking information on how to disclose to sexual partners.

The lowest ranked US site (103/113) was the Florida-based dabtheaidsbearproject.com ("An American journey of hope"), a grassroots, multi-media website with photographs of AIDS bears ("Angel Bears") and their human friends. The graphics were accompanied by a description of the bears' origin as symbols of comfort during a time when HIV was a certain death sentence. On the homepage, messages of hope and self-empowerment offered a warm welcome to HIV-infected people and friends. However, this friendliness was offset by a stern warning about non-disclosure being both immoral and a felony in most states and a 3,500-word legal section which threatened search engines with legal action if they used algorithms, spyware, and other tracking devices for commercial or other purposes. Although Google's search-and-store method of classifying data probably determined the website's Internet ranking, the threatening tone of the legal section might also have contributed to the low priority score in Table 1.

Value rankings

Table 1 lists the V. Score on quality of advice. The V. Scores ranged from 1 (least helpful) to 5 (most helpful) and bore little relation to Google's priority rankings. For instance, the top ranked U.S. site (AIDSmeds.com) provided a cursory 10 lines of information for a score of 2. The second-ranked site (Thewellproject.com, a women's resource network) also earned a score of 2 for 10 lines of grimly worded text on the legal consequences of non-disclosure. The third ranked site (Thebody.com) provided comprehensive and up-to-date information for a score of 4, but the fourth ranked site (Webmed.com) offered a meager two lines for a score of 1(the advice was less helpful than in the lowest-ranked U.S. site). Most remaining websites did not originate in the United States.

Foreign websites earned higher quality scores than U.S. websites. Sites in the United Kingdom, Canada, and Australia provided detailed legal information (e.g., explanations about the difference between reckless and intentional transmission in U.K. law), as well as advice on how to disclose to sexual partners in keeping with the law. These sites were often affiliated with government agencies and had benefited from the expertise that agency personnel provided to community-based organizations as a public service. Most of these sites catered to particular audiences or communities. To illustrate, Gmfa.org.uk (Gay Men Fight AIDS in the United Kingdom) offered expert advice on HIV disclosure and the law in accessible language ending with the gentle reminder to "take responsibility for your own health and safety when having sex." In keeping with its mission for advocacy and self-empowerment, the website lamented the trend toward criminalization – which it deemed ineffective -- and provided a link to an affiliate that advocated for legal change. In contrast to the U.S. sites, Black men were depicted in almost every image on the homepage and links, suggesting that the writers took account of HIV statistics involving men of color and had tailored their message accordingly.

The Body.com (a site for HIV-infected people) provided high quality advice for HIV-infected people, which helped to support the site's self-proclaimed position as "the largest HIV/AIDS resource on the net." Webpage authors offered friendly advice, which occasionally challenged the criminalization of HIV. For example, in a column titled "Sex While HIV Positive: The New Criminals," the writer had advice on how to obtain proof of disclosure and expressed doubt about the wisdom of criminalization by stating: "[T]he more I have learned about the criminalization of HIV non-disclosure, the more I am convinced these laws are applied badly and actually do more harm than good. If I don't get tested, I can't be prosecuted for not disclosing my status, right?" An accompanying video blog discussed the fear of people being tested because of criminalization, which led to forgoing life-saving drugs that would also prevent HIV transmission. By contrast, few of the other U.S. websites went into such detail, with most advice consisting of simple directives to disclose to sexual partners as a moral and legal necessity.

How useful is the US advice?

Narratives on HIV disclosure and the law can help Internet users to resolve the legal aspects of safer-sex, that is, sexual activity within the law. Table Two summarizes advice on HIV disclosure and the law in top ranked U.S. websites; that is, the 10 sites that were most likely to be read by Internet users seeking advice on disclosure to sexual partners.

All ten sites emphasized the basic importance of complying with the law. Once again, the amount of advice varied widely with the most complete information appearing on Thebody.com. A webpage titled: "Should you disclose?" sounded a cautionary note, followed by statements such as: "Many of these laws were written early in the epidemic, and were fear driven... . Deciding who should be punished, and for what offense, often lies in the hands of politicians and court systems that base their decisions on old data and personal prejudices." The site defined willful exposure according to California law, explained how non-disclosure could lead to both criminal and civil penalties, and urged readers to disclose their HIV status in order to avoid the risk of prosecution. Links to other web pages led to advice on how to obtain proof of disclosure, including this nugget of wisdom: "You can share your status before you meet your date in person, such as over the Internet, or in a print personal ad, after a few preliminary dates when you know you'd like to pursue the relationship further." Personal anecdotes helped to frame the importance of disclosure. For example: "For Tracy Johnson, 22 and HIV-positive, romance often begins at a karaoke bar. There's music, conversation and innocent touching. He's at ease until it's time for the first kiss -- that's when he leans in, pulls out the document and asks the object of his affection to sign, indicating he's shared that he has HIV. That piece of paper, he believes, could save him from years behind bars if a partner ever alleges that he didn't disclose his status. He carries it everywhere."

Table 2. Disclosure+law content in top 10 U.S. websites

No 1. Aidsmeds.com, No. 5, Mdjunction.com (10 lines)

"It's important for you to be aware of what the laws are in your state with regard to *contract tracing* and *partner notification.* Contact tracing refers to the efforts of government agencies to identify any and all persons who might be at risk of contracting HIV from an infected person. Partner notification refers to information conveyed to spouses, sexual partners, needle sharers and others who might be at risk for HIV infection. The laws regarding this vary from state to state. In many states, partner notification can be done anonymously through the state's Department of Health. The Department of Health in your state is a good source of information about what the legal procedure is in your state and how it might apply to you."

No 2. Thewellproject.com (10 lines)

"In most cases, sharing your HIV status is a personal choice, but in the case of sexual relationships, it can be a legal requirement. It is best if you disclose your status prior to having sex with anyone new. Non-disclosure of HIV status in a sexual relationship can lead to criminal charges whether or not your partner becomes infected with HIV. In most states, the law requires that you disclose your HIV status before knowingly exposing or transmitting HIV to someone else. Penalties vary from state to state. In many states, you can be found guilty of a felony for not telling a sexual partner you are HIV+ before having intimate contact."

No 3. TheBody.Com (43 lines, multiple links, e-card: 15 lines of text excerpted below)

"Currently about 27 [sic] states have established criminal penalties for knowingly exposing or transmitting HIV to someone else. In California, the "Willful Exposure" law (although narrowly written and difficult to prosecute) makes exposing someone else to HIV (whether they become infected or not) a felony punishable by up to eight years in prison. In Alabama, you can be prosecuted for "Conducting yourself in manner likely to transmit the disease." (Just the thought of that is scary) ... If you tell the other person that you have HIV before insertion, you cannot be prosecuted criminally. It would have to be proven in court that you had "specific intent" to infect the other person in order to be prosecuted criminally. In a civil case, the specifics to which you could be found guilty are much more flexible -- so be careful. Check with your local ASO (AIDS Service Organization) or legal services to find out what the laws are in your area."

No 4. WebmMD.com, No. 6, Friendsofaids.org (2 lines, e-card)

"State laws make it illegal to knowingly infect others. If you have unprotected sex without telling others, you're putting yourself at legal risk, as well as endangering the health of your partners."

No 7. Poz.Com (7 lines, multiple links, e-card)

"Bear in mind that sometimes you are legally required to disclose to a sexual partner. Many states have laws that make it illegal to transmit HIV or to have unprotected sex without telling your partner your status. Don't panic: Prosecutions are relatively rare because prosecutors usually have to prove that the person with HIV intended to infect his or her partner, which isn't easy. To find out if your state has a criminalization law on the books, visit www.lambdalegal.org."

No 8. Ehow.com (32 lines, e-card: 10 lines of text excerpted below)

"There are some circumstances in which it is legal for others to disclose [your HIV status], but this is only in very specific circumstances. 1. *Willful Exposure:* Willful exposure happens when someone knows she has HIV and does not disclose to sex partners and is not mindful of the possible transmission. Several states have passed laws to treat willful exposure as a criminal offense. 2. *Criminalization:* Many states have laws in place to criminalize willful exposure, and in the history of the disease, at least 300 people have been criminally prosecuted for knowingly infecting others. Depending on the state, the crime can be as severe as manslaughter or attempted manslaughter charge."

No 9. Doh.state.fl.org (13 lines, e-card)

"Discussing and disclosing HIV status is a two-way street. Be it right or wrong, most people feel that when a person knows that he/she is HIV+ then he/she has an obligation to tell the other person, and counselors are encouraged to help people with this process. Also, laws in some areas require disclosure of HIV+ status prior to sex. However, both partners should be responsible for knowing their own status, disclosing their own status when it seems important, and asking their partner about their status if they want to know. There is debate around whether partners have a right to know if their partner is HIV+, in order to be able to make a fully informed decision about what sexual behavior to engage in. Some HIV+ persons believe that if they only have protected sex, there is no need for disclosure, especially with casual partners, and that encouraging disclosure only serves to further stigmatize HIV+ persons. These issues can be complicated by complex gender role norms and local laws—23 [sic] states have laws that make it a crime for a person to engage in certain risk behaviors without disclosing their HIV status."

No 10. Wdxcyber.com (2 lines)

"It is important to note that you are obliged to tell your partner about your status before any sexual activity occurs. In some US states, this is the law."

A photograph of an African American man accompanied the text - the first such image to appear on any of the top U.S. sites in relation to HIV disclosure.

The middle ground for advice was occupied by websites such as the Florida Department of Health's Dohfla.org, the HIV advocacy website Poz.com, and eHow.com, a general advice website. These sites offered formal advice on HIV disclosure and the law as well as a link to inSpot.org for partner notification. InSpot is a sexual health site that allows people with STIs to notify partners by sending an anonymous e-card to the recipient's address. The site has a variety of messages to suit the sender's style, gender, or type of sexual encounter. Two of these messages read: "I got diagnosed with an STD and you might have been exposed. Get checked out" and more explicitly, "I got screwed while screwing, you might have too." The e-card option guaranteed anonymity for the sender but lacked hardcopies that could be printed out for proof of disclosure.

With ten lines of primary text, eHow.com was the most informative of the intermediate sites in defining willful exposure as a crime, discussing state laws, and providing a link to inSpot. Two intermediate sites (Aidsmeds.com and Mdjunction.com) offered identical advice, which consisted of advising users to contact their respective health departments. With ten lines of advice, Thewellproject.com advised readers that disclosure of a positive HIV diagnosis to sexual partners was a legal requirement, and that non-disclosure was a felony crime in many states. Despite being a California-based health resource for women, the site did not have advice on legal issues facing California women, such as mandatory HIV testing of sex workers, laws that target female sex workers for criminal non-disclosure, and prosecutions that frame HIV-infected women as prostitutes.

The least helpful sites also provided few lines of text. For example, with only two lines on HIV disclosure and the law apiece, the women's resource siteWdxcyber.com, the HIV advocacy site Friendsofaids.org, and the general medical website Webmd.com were the least explanatory of all websites in the sample. These forums issued a formal warning about the risks of prosecution without useful tips on how to disclose in order to avoid legal trouble. Elaboration would have helped Internet users to understand the legal complexities of non-disclosure, especially on questions such as: Is "knowingly" the same as "intentionally?" Does kissing or oral sex count as sex for legal purposes? How do I avoid being rejected, injured, or "outed" if I disclose?

It is worth reiterating that the highly ranked US websites were not always the best sources for information on disclosure and the law. Some lower-ranked sites were more informative but were too far down the list to be read by most Internet users. Some overseas sites were excellent purveyors of advice even if their legal sections were too parochial for U.S. use. For example, the Canadian website Positiveside.ca advised users about obtaining proof of disclosure by inviting a friend, medical provider, or counselor to be present during the act of disclosure (e.g., by taking the disclosee to a doctor's appointment) or by keeping written evidence of disclosure from the Internet or in a personal diary in order to prevent any he said/he said scenarios in court. The text was accompanied by an image of a naked man in handcuffs and a warning that: "Even if you told a person before sex that you are HIV positive, the person might lie and say that you did not. Judges and juries have decided many of the legal cases about HIV, sex and disclosure based on credibility – whom they believed or didn't believe. In a court case, it is important to have evidence to show that you disclosed and that the other person knew your HIV status."

Whose responsibility?

Advice on U.S. websites was often brief and legalistic (e.g., "State laws make it illegal to knowingly infect others") with an explicit emphasis on individual responsibility. Some advocacy sites had conflicting advice on whether or not to follow U.S. law for disclosing a positive HIV diagnosis to sexual partners. For example, ambivalence toward the law was evident in this text from Aidsmeds.com: "For those who are single and are HIV positive, if and when to disclose can be addressed in different ways. Some people prefer to get the issue out into the open immediately. Others prefer to wait and see if the relationship is going to develop beyond a first date or casual dating. Still others feel that as long they're having safer sex, the risk is minimal to the other person, so why even bring the subject up?" The site offered a stepwise process to calculate the risk of rejection but fell short on offering helpful tips about how to disclose, obtain proof of disclosure, and avoid "he said/she said" scenarios that could end in litigation.

Conflicting advice sometimes appeared on web pages and links that were authored by different people over a period of years. Taking Thebody.com as an example, a 2002 item titled "Should you disclose your HIV status to a potential sexual partner?" offered timely warnings about criminalization while also stating: "Disclosure is not easy for everyone, and in certain situations is not an option (such as where disclosing could cause physical injury to yourself)." By 2011, sites such as Poz.com and Thebody.com had abandoned this position, adopted a defensive tone over the proliferation of HIV-specific laws, and urged members to watch out for potential legal problems. This stance appeared in statements such as: "I guess we should all start making any sexual partners [use a condom] or sign a consent form saying they understand the risks" (Poz.com), and: "Most of us are caring, law-abiding human beings who want to be good citizens. So we're stuck in that rock and hard place where we have to figure out, 'How do I prove I didn't break that law?' ... It really is bizarre what we have to go through to protect ourselves" (Thebody.com). The legal mandate of individual responsibility was certainly irksome to some people who had shouldered the burden of disclosure from the outset. An advocate protested: "Given this new reality [the effectiveness of ARV drugs in reducing HIV transmission], I am reconsidering my options. [F]or once it would be nice if my prospective partners took responsibility for their own health and asked me if I had HIV so that I wouldn't have to carry the burden of telling them first" (Vanessa Johnson, Thebody.com). This defiance was tempered by surrender to U.S. law and regret that the mutual responsibility model had never appeared to be a viable option.

Websites that advocated mutual responsibility were fewer in number. The U.K site International Planned Parenthood Fund (IPPF.org) was a notable exception. In the 2010 report Happy, Healthy and Hot, the IPPF [43] took a bold stand by stating: "Young people living with HIV have the right to decide if, when, and how to disclose their HIV status" (p. 3), and further, "Some countries have laws that violate the right of young people living with HIV to decide whether to disclose or face the possibility of criminal charges" (p. 6). These statements provoked outrage from conservative websites such as Concerned Women for America (CWFA.org) and Red State (Redstate.com), which complained of radical extremism and hippy sensibilities from the 1970s. On Poz.com, the opening salvo of a U.S-European forum also hinted at opposition to the individual responsibility model for disclosure. Here, the convener challenged the panel by asking: "Who's responsible for new infections? Criminalization says it's the [Person with AIDS]. Prevention says both partners. Right now, criminalization is winning." The cultural divide between Europeans and the U.S. was revealed in vigorous discussions about the rights and wrongs of criminalization for non-disclosure, especially in prosecuting Black men "for having sex with White women... . The case of Nushawn Williams is like a dark cloud hanging over this whole discussion." This flashpoint was evident in statements about criminalization being punitive and "useless" for HIV prevention (Europe) compared to being "inevitable" or "just retribution" for a wronged partner (U.S.). Even among advocates on the panel, the shared responsibility model was being debated in relation to disclosure and U.S. law.

Discussion

The results of this study indicate that highly ranked websites (i.e., medical or HIV sites that attract large audiences) are more likely to be consulted than sites that appear lower in the ranking hierarchy. This finding has implications for the accessibility of Internet advice on HIV disclosure and the law. First, information on the legal aspects of disclosure was missing from one third of the top ranked websites, suggesting that Internet users might be poorly served when they seek critical advice on disclosure in an era of HIV criminalization. Second, the quality of advice from these websites did not match their priority rankings. For example, the well-known U.S. POZ.com (an advocacy website), which offered advice from a friendly, consumer-oriented perspective, earned a lower Google ranking than suggested by the popularity of POZ magazine, a waiting room staple in HIV clinics in the United States.

The discrepancy between quality of information and ranking score highlights a growing problem for Internet searches in the age of personalization. Unless users enter a web address themselves, then they are beholden to search engines that prioritize sites according to popularity (the highest number of hits) and commercial value (advertising links), and also to websites that use metatags to increase their visibility [42]. Google's ranking algorithm tailors Internet results according to a user's search history so that retrievals can vary greatly from one person or computer to another. Another complicating factor is that Internet searches produce an abundance of media stories, scientific articles, legal caches, blogs, and sundry posts on HIV disclosure and the law; in other words, a surfeit of information that has to be sifted through in order to reach the desired destination. This abundance is not only eye opening but also instructive about the risks of prosecution for HIV-related offenses. For example, the present author's searches for websites on HIV disclosure produced media headlines such as "Man charged with failing to disclose HIV status to partner," "Man charged with murder for spreading HIV," and "Iowa man sentenced to 25 years in prison for failure to disclose." These results were as ubiquitous as they were alarming and served as a clarion call to Internet users about the risks of non-disclosure.

The lack of information on HIV disclosure and the law on many U.S. websites can be compared to the comprehensive information on sites in the U.K., Australia, and Canada. The brevity of U.S. advice on the legal aspects of HIV disclosure was also at odds with the amount of advice on other HIV-related topics on the U.S. sites, including when and how to disclose to family members. One explanation for the deficit of legal information relates to the practical difficulties of addressing the legal background of 50 states that have diverse criminal codes and statutes for non-disclosure as a crime. Although the problem could easily be remedied by providing a link to each state's HIV laws, most U.S. sites avoided the issue by referring users to state health departments or by making brief statements about non-disclosure as a crime. Websites from countries with a single legal system (e.g., England, Canada, Australia) did not encounter this problem. Users in these countries generally have greater access to official information and expertise provided specifically for HIV-related websites. However, the issue of quality is a vexed one for the Internet regardless of mitigating factors such as a country's system of laws or integrated advice. Purcell, Wilson, and Delamothe [44] noted that many popular websites fail to satisfy the informational needs of users who seek advice for health problems, a troubling finding when health consumers are expected to be both proactive and self-empowered in the Internet age [45].

Internet users are often portrayed as self-empowered seekers of information. However, the ideal of self-empowerment can be difficult to achieve when it comes to eliciting information about a partner's STI history [46]. Although the proactive approach to information seeking was the basis for the mutual responsibility model for HIV prevention in the 1980s, the present study found that present models of information-sharing were uni-directional – from HIV-infected people to their sexual partners – as required by U.S. law. One caveat to this finding was that advocacy-minded U.S. websites tended to advise HIV-infected people to obtain proof of disclosure to guard against prosecution in contested cases. The fact that most websites in the present study fully endorsed the individual responsibility model for HIV-infected users suggests a natural evolution of events in terms of public sentiment and the law - a trend recently bolstered by CDC policies to ensure that HIV-infected people disclose to sexual partners [47]. Despite this evolution, the ambivalence of some websites suggests that advocates have not endorsed fully the flight from mutual responsibility or accepted the legal premise that non-disclosure is responsible for spreading HIV.

The present study found one-size-fits-all advice on many U.S. sites. This uniformity neglected the special risks of prosecution for African Americans who are HIV-infected in disproportionate numbers compared to other citizens. Research by Stein et al. [48] found that Black men were over three times less likely to disclose to sexual partners than Whites and Hispanics and were twice as reluctant as Black women to do so. In the United Kingdom, Elford et al. [49] reported that Africans were significantly less likely than gay men to disclose to sexual partners about being HIV-infected. The Serovich et al. [40] study of HIV disclosure patterns found that non-disclosure rates were high (<50%) regardless of racial differences, and that the act of disclosure is difficult and socially fraught for many people. African American men's avoidance of disclosure may account, in part, for racial disparities in criminal prosecutions for HIV-related crimes although the reverse might also be true: Black men, who are historically portrayed in terms of a "monstrous masculinity" [3] might be reluctant to disclose if they fear being targeted for prosecution by health officials and the police. Such men need tailored advice on how to disclose, why they should disclose, and how to obtain proof of disclosure in order to avoid prosecution. It is possible that such advice is being delivered at time of diagnosis or in informal or community forums. However, the men's reluctance to disclose as identified by Stein et al [48] and even greater reluctance to be tested for HIV as evident from "take the test, risk arrest" warnings that circulate among African American men [50], suggest that the anonymity of the Internet could be useful for reaching this audience, and for providing life-saving information that is also an "insurance policy" against prosecution.

Finally, there is the question of where HIV-infected people are likely to seek advice for disclosure. As noted, HIV-infected people are usually counseled in a health setting at the time of their initial diagnosis. This counseling might be followed up by additional advice on HIV disclosure at the same site at a later date. However, it is difficult to remember advice being delivered in highly emotionally charged situations, and a significant proportion of HIV-infected people are lost to follow-up care after being diagnosed [51]. It is here that the Internet can fill an important role in providing supplementary information on HIV disclosure and the law, and it is imperative that excellent, post-diagnosis advice is available for people who seek anonymity while coming to terms with a life-changing condition. The advice should, at a minimum, provide a confidential helpline for Internet users who fear being prosecuted for non-disclosure, links to information on relevant laws of their state, and also offer e-referrals to legal professionals or local AIDS service agency employees who could then explain these laws in detail.

The findings of this study should be interpreted with caution. It is possible that the Internet searches yielded data that would be different if performed at a different time and place. The search engine's personalized algorithm guarantees that Internet results always will be somewhat idiosyncratic, although the results presented here were generated from four different computers in an effort to avoid this problem. Second, the searches generated hundreds of pages of results that had to be culled carefully, sorted, labeled, and then cross-identified. It is unlikely that a typical individual would take the same trouble to identify relevant advice on HIV disclosure and the law. Third, there is the danger of subjective judgments about the quality of advice, especially in a sole-rater content analysis. In order to avoid this problem, the present author compared the data in each category in a reiterative, line-by-line basis until satisfied that the scores were distributed fairly. However, it should be acknowledged that the sole-rater content analysis is a limitation of the study, and that an inter-rater system would have enhanced the reliability of the results.

The social science implications of the present study are threefold. First, racial differences and race-based stereotyping, especially as they pertain to stigma and HIV serostatus disclosure, present a challenge for public health goals to expand HIV testing [52]. The results presented here suggest that African American men, who are often targeted for prosecution, have little access to culturally-relevant information on the why, where, when, and how of disclosure, or to dedicated websites that promote their legal rights while also advocating HIV testing to protect their own and their partners' health. This deficit should be addressed as a matter of urgency. Second, the lack of culturally relevant information, together with media hyperbole about cases involving African American men, are likely to stymie national goals for expanded HIV testing. If Internet users are exposed to sensational media reports, and if website information is lacking or consists mainly of terse "it's the law" declarations, then users are likely to become more fearful than informed about the topic. U.S. websites should address disclosure and the law in friendly, personalized terms in order to empower people to disclose to sexual partners while ensuring their own safety in potentially awkward, perhaps dangerous situations. Following the Canadian, U.K., and Australian models, this information could come from a central clearing house that provides accurate, consistent, and well written material as a public service. Third, the present study highlighted how HIV stigma drove U.S. legal policy, more recently in relation to minority ethnic status. Since multiple stigmas affect the most vulnerable populations, and HIV criminalization has gathered pace in recent years, community websites could make a better effort at offering tailored advice for at-risk populations, and could also engage in legal advocacy to help reduce the stigma of being HIV-infected as presently conceived in U.S. law.

References

[1] Bennett-Carlson R, Faria D, Hanssens C. Positive Justice Project: Ending and defending against HIV criminalization. *A manual for advocates.* Volume 1. New York, NY: Center HIV Law Policy, 2010. Accessed 2011 June 12. URL: http://www.hivlawandpolicy.org/resources/view/564.

[2] Treichler PA. *How to have theory in an epidemic: Cultural chronicles of AIDS.* Durham, NC: Duke University Press, 1999.

[3] Strub S. *Prevention vs. prosecution: Creating a viral underclass,* 2011. Accessed 2011 Oct 28. URL: http://blogs.poz.com/sean/archives/2011/10/prevention_vs_prosec.html.

[4] Persson A, Newman C. Making monsters: Crime and race in recent Western media coverage of HIV. *Soc Health Illness* 2008;30:632-46.

[5] Bernard E. *Prosecutions for HIV exposure and transmission on the rise throughout Europe.* Accessed 2011 Jul 27.URL: http://www.aidsmap.com/en/news9/9FFE7E7EA6-2E16-4376-8FC4-A8E82B6325A2.asp

[6] Pebody R. North America and Western Europe lead the world in criminalising HIV transmission and exposure. *XVIII International AIDS Conference,* Vienna, Austria, 2010. Accessed 2011 Jul 22. URL: http://www.aidsmap.com/North-America-and-Western-Europe-lead-the-world-in-criminalising-HIV-transmission-and-exposure/page/1447653/

[7] Lahey KE. The new line of defense: Criminal HIV transmission laws. *Syracuse J Legis Pol* 1995;1:85-95.

[8] Lazzarini Z, Bray S, Burris, S. Evaluating the impact of criminal laws on HIV risk behavior. *J Laws Med Ethics* 2002;30(2):239-53.

[9] Krom D. HIV-specific knowing transmission statutes: A proposal to help fight an epidemic. *St John's J Leg Comm* 1999;14:253-78.

[10] Canadian HIV/AIDS Legal Network, 2011. *Criminal law and HIV.* Accessed 2011 Jul 30. URL: http://library.catie.ca/PDF/ATI-10000s/18149.pdf.

[11] Bennett-Carlson R, Faria D, Hanssens C. *Positive Justice Project: Prosecutions and arrests for HIV exposure in the United States,* 2008-2011. New York, NY: The Center for HIV Law and Policy, 2011. Accessed 2011 Aug 20. URL: http://www.hivlawandpolicy.org/resources/view/456.

[12] Homeland Security Newswire. *HIV positive Michigan man fights bioterrorism charge after allegedly biting neighbor,* 2010. Accessed 2011 Jul 12. URL: http://homelandsecuritynewswire.com/hiv-positive-michigan-man-fights-bioterrorism-charge-after-allegedly-biting-neighbor.

[13] Bickerstaff E. *HIV and the media in the US.* Impact:12 (February). UK: National AIDS Trust, 2007.

[14] Del Amo J, Carol AM, Martinez C, Field V, Broring, G. *HIV/AIDS and migration in European printed media: An analysis of daily newspapers. Brussels,* Belgium: AIDS and Mobility Working Group, 2006. Accessed 2011 May 7. URL: http://ws5.evision.nl/systeem3/images/final%20report%20version%207%20november.pdf.

[15] Koop CE. *Surgeon General's report on acquired immune deficiency syndrome*. Washington DC: Public Health Service, 1986.

[16] Cochran SE, Mays VM. Sex, lies, and HIV. N Engl J Med 1990;322:774-775.

[17] Offer C, Grinstead O, Goldstein E, Mamary E, Alvarado N, Euren J, et al. Responsibility for HIV prevention: Patterns of attribution among HIV-seropositive gay and bisexual men. *AIDS Educ Prev* 2007;19(1):24-35.

[18] Wingood GM, DiClemente RJ. The effects of an abusive primary partner on the condom use and sexual negotiation practices of African-American women. *Am J Pub Health* 1997;87(6):1016-8.

[19] Duffin R. *Serostatus, risk and responsibility. New South Wales Department of Health,* 2004. Accessed 2011 November 7. URL: http://www.sprc.unsw.edu.au/media/File/SRB06.pdf.

[20] Bayer R. AIDS prevention – Sexual ethics and responsibility. *N Engl J Med* 1996;334:1540-2.

[21] National Institute of Allergy and Infectious Diseases. *HIV/AIDS: Treatment of HIV infection.* Washington, DC: U.S. Dept Health Human Serv, 2009. Accessed 2011 Aug 1. URL:http://www.niaid.nih.gov/topics/hivaids/understanding/treatment/pages/default.aspx.

[22] Donnell D, Baeten JM, Kiarie J, Thomas KK, Stevens W, Cohen CR et al. Heterosexual HIV-1 transmission after initiation of antiretroviral therapy: A prospective cohort analysis. *Lancet* 2010;375(9731):2092-8.

[23] Centers for Disease Control and Prevention. *Advancing HIV Prevention: Progress Summary,* 2003-2005. Atlanta, GA: Nat Cent HIV/AIDS Vir Hep STDTB Prev, 2005.Accessed 2011 Jun 19. URL: http://www.cdc.gov/hiv/topics/prev_prog/AHP/resources/factsheets/pdf/Progress_2005.pdf.

[24] Centers for Disease Control and Prevention. Hepatitis C information for the public. Atlanta, GA: *Nat Cent HIV/AIDS,* Vir Hep STD TB Prevention, 2008. Accessed 2011 Jul 10: URL: http://www.cdc.gov/hepatitis/C/cFAQ.htm.

[25] Hepatitis B Foundation. *General Information.* Accessed 2011 Jun 30. URL: http://www.hepb.org/patients/general_information.htm.

[26] James R. A review of HIV transmission and exposure cases in Australia, the United Kingdom, Sweden and Switzerland. *Int AIDS Soc Conf, Vienna,* Austria, 2010. Accessed 2011 Oct 26. URL: http://birkbeck.academia.edu/MatthewWeait/Papers/219944/Who_Gets_Prosecuted.

[27] Karon JM, Fleming, PL, Steketee RW, De Cock KM. HIV in the United States at the turn of the century: An epidemic in transition. *Am J Pub Health* 2001;91(7):1060-8.

[28] The Henry J. Kaiser Family Foundation. *Black Americans and AIDS,* 2007. Accessed 2011 Oct 28. URL:http://www.kff.org/hivaids/upload/6089-04.pdf.

[29] Rosenberg SD, Goodman, LA, Osher, FC, Swarz MS, Essock SM, Butterfield MI et al. Prevalence of HIV, hepatitis B, and hepatitis C in people with severe mental illness. *Am J Pub Health* 2001;91(1):31-37.

[30] Mykhalovskiy E, Betteridge G, McLay D. *HIV non-disclosure and the criminal law: Establishing policy options for Ontario,* Toronto. Toronto, CA: Canada's AIDS Treatment Information Exchange, 2010. Accessed 2011 Aug 1. URL: http://www.catie.ca/pdf/Brochures/HIV-non-disclosure-criminal-law.pdf.

[31] Worth H, Patton C, Goldstein D. Reckless vectors: The infecting 'Other' in HIV/AIDS law. *Sex Res Soc Pol* 2005;2(2):3-14.

[32] Wnuk D, Chapman JE, Jeglic EL. Development and refinement of a measure of attitudes toward sex offender treatment. *J Off Rehab* 2006;43(3):35-47.

[33] Heath L. Mass media and fear of crime. *Am Behav Sci* 1996;39(4):379-386.

[34] Lichtenstein B. *Social stigma in the sexual epidemics: Dangerous Dynamics. CO*: Lynne Reiner Publishers, 2012.

[35] Kenney SV. Criminalizing HIV transmission: Lessons learned from history and a model for the future. *J Cont Law Pol* 1992;8:245-73.

[36] Merminod A. The deterrence rationale in the criminalization of HIV/AIDS. *Lex Electr,* 2009;13:3.Accessed 2011 Jul 10. URL: http://www.lexelectronica.org/docs/articles_226.pdf.

[37] Shouse RL, Kajese T, Hall HI, Valleroy LA.Late HIV Testing – 34 states, 1996-2005. *Morb Mort Week Rep,* 2009;58(24):661-65.

[38] Centers for Disease Control and Prevention. *HIV in the United States: An overview.* Atlanta, GA: Nat Cent HIV/AIDS Vir Hep STD TB Prev, 2010. Accessed 2011 Jul 12. URL: http://www.cdc.gov/hiv/topics/surveillance/resources/factsheets/us_overview.htm

[39] Galletly CL, Pinkerton SD. Conflicting messages: How criminal HIV disclosure laws undermine public health efforts to control the spread of HIV. *AIDS Behav* 2006;10: 451-61.

[40] Serovich JE, Mosack KE. Reasons for HIV disclosure or nondisclosure to casual sexual partners. *AIDS Educ Prev* 2003;15(1):70-80.

[41] Grossman HP, Guillory AK. Law trends and news. Washington, DC: *AmBar Assoc,* 2004. Accessed 2011 Jul 7. URL: http://www.americanbar.org/content/newsletter/publications/law_trends_news_practice_area_e_newsletter_home/hipaa.html.

[42] Pariser, E. *The filter bubble: What the internet is hiding from you.* New York, NY: Penguin, 2011.

[43] International Planned Parenthood Federation. *Healthy, happy, and hot: A young person's guide to their rights, sexuality and living with HIV.* Accessed 2011 July 21. URL:http://www.ippf.org/NR/rdonlyres/B4462DDE-487D-4194-B0E0-193A04095819/0/HappyHealthyHot.pdf.

[44] Purcell GP, Wilson P, Delamothe T. The quality of health information on the internet: As for any other medium it varies widely: Regulation is not the answer. *BMJ* 2002;324(7337):557-8.

[45] Lewis, T. Seeking health information on the internet: Lifestyle choice or bad attack of cyberchrondria? *Med Cult Soc* 2006;28(4):521-39.

[46] Wolitski RJ, Bailey CJ, O'Leary A, Gomez CA, Parsons JT. Self-perceived responsibility of HIV-seropositive men who have sex with men for preventing HIV transmission. *AIDS Behav* 2003;7(4):363-72.

[47] Gorbach PM, Galea JT, Amani B, Shin A, Celum C, Golden MR. Don't ask, don't tell: Patterns of HIV disclosure among HIV positive men who have sex with men with recent STI practicing high risk behaviour in Los Angeles and Seattle. *Sex Trans Dis* 2004;80: 512-7.

[48] Stein MD, Freedberg KA, Sullivan LM, Savetsky J, Levenson SM, Hingson R, et al. Disclosure of HIV status to sexual partners. *Arch Int Med* 1998;158:253-57.

[49] Elford J, Ibrahim F, Bukutu C, Anderson J. Disclosure of HIV status: The role of ethnicity among people living with HIV in London. *J Acquir Immune Defic Syndr* 2008;47:514-21.

[50] Lichtenstein B. *Overcoming Stigma. National Harbor,* MD: NatSummit HIV Diag Prev Access Care, 2010.

[51] Cairns G. *London patient surveys find widely different rates of patients referred to care and lost to follow-up,* 2009. Accessed 2011 Jul 12. URL: http://www.aidsmap.com/London-patient-surveys-find-widely-different-rates-of-patients-referred-to-care-and-lost-to-follow-up/page/1434061/.

[52] The White House Office of National AIDS Policy. *National HIV/AIDS Strategy for the United States,* 2010. Accessed 2011 Nov 1. URL: http://www.whitehouse.gov/sites/default/files/uploads/NHAS.pdf.

In: Human Immunodeficiency Virus …
Editors: Hugh Klein and Joav Merrick

ISBN: 978-1-62081-293-8

Chapter III

Childhood maltreatment and HIV risk-taking among men using the internet specifically to find partners for unprotected sex

Hugh Klein*[*1,2] and David Tilley[3]
[1]Kensington Research Institute, Silver Spring, Maryland
[2]Prevention Sciences Research Center, Morgan State University, Baltimore, Maryland
[3]Department of Community and Family Health, University of South Florida, Tampa, Florida, US

Abstract

Using a Syndemics Theory conceptual model, this study examines the relationship between childhood maltreatment experiences and involvement in HIV risk taking in a sample of adult men who actively seek partners for unprotected sex via the Internet. The study was based on a national random sample of 332 men who have sex with men (MSM), who use the Internet to seek men with whom they can engage in unprotected sex. Data collection was conducted via telephone interviews between January 2008 and May 2009. Structural equation analysis was undertaken to examine the specific nature of the relationships involved in understanding HIV risk practices. Childhood maltreatment experiences were not found to be related directly to involvement in HIV risk taking in adulthood. Childhood maltreatment, particularly in the form of emotional neglect, was found to be an important variable in the overall structural equation. Its effect on HIV risk taking was indirect, operating principally by having a negative impact upon self-esteem, which in turn had a negative effect on attitudes toward condom use, which in turn were related strongly and directly to risk taking. We conclude that childhood maltreatment experiences are relevant to understanding HIV risk practices among MSM in adulthood,

* Correspondence: Hugh Klein, PhD, Kensington Research Institute, 401 Schuyler Road, Silver Spring, Maryland 20910, USA. E-mail: hughk@aol.com (primary) or hughkhughk@yahoo.com (secondary).

but the relationship is not as simple as usually conceptualized. Rather, childhood maltreatment appears to impact risk taking indirectly, through its effects on mental health functioning, which in turn affects risk-related attitudes.

Introduction

Childhood maltreatment, whether in the form of sexual abuse, physical abuse, emotional abuse, or neglect, has been linked with a wide variety of adverse outcomes in adulthood. These include, among others, mental health problems (e.g., depression, anxiety, post-traumatic stress disorder, attempted suicide, history of substance abuse) [1], HIV risk behaviors [2,3], and obesity [4]. This has been true for a number of populations, including men who have sex with men [3,5], heterosexual men [6], lesbians [4], and heterosexual women [2], indicating that the effects of early-life maltreatment are far-reaching and long-lasting.

Sexual abuse experiences have been linked with a greater risk for practicing risky sex later in life in men who have sex with men (MSM), specifically because of the effect of these experiences on men's psychological health. Childhood sexual abuse was discussed as a precursor to adulthood involvement in HIV risk-taking in Fields, Malebranche, and Feist-Price's [7] research on African American MSM. Catania and colleagues [8: 925] noted that childhood sexual abuse "contributes to the ongoing HIV epidemic among MSM by distorting or undermining critical motivational, coping, and interpersonal factors that, in turn, influence adult sexual risk behavior." Dorais' [5] qualitative study of childhood sexual abuse and HIV risk taking among MSM revealed the former to be associated with an inability to assert oneself with regard to one's sexual safety and a greater tendency toward sexual compulsivity. In their bi-coastal study of HIV-positive MSM, O'Leary, Purcell, Remien, and Gomez [9] reported a link between childhood sexual abuse and engaging in unprotected anal intercourse with serodiscordant partners. In a study of gay and bisexual men attending a midwestern gay pride festival, childhood sexual abuse was found to be related to the likelihood of being HIV-positive, having exchanged sex for money, and the use of sex-related drugs, but not to the practice of unprotected sex [10]. In another study of men attending a different city's gay pride festival [11], childhood sexual abuse was found to be related to a history of exchanging sex for drugs and/or money, but not to unprotected anal intercourse. Saewyc and colleagues [12] studied adolescents located in the Pacific Northwest, and concluded that sexual victimization contributed to greater overall HIV risk behavior involvement (based on a composite scale measuring seven different HIV risk practices) among the gay and bisexual students in their sample. Rosario, Schrimshaw, and Hunter [13] also based their work on gay and bisexual adolescents and young adults, and found that childhood sexual abuse was related to having a larger number of sex partners, which in turn was related to a greater likelihood of engaging in unprotected anal sex.

In contrast to the preceding, the present authors find it noteworthy that studies examining the effects of other types of childhood maltreatment (e.g., physical abuse, emotional abuse, emotional neglect, physical neglect) on HIV risk taking are very scarce in the published literature. One noteworthy exception is the research conducted by Paul, Catania, Pollack, and Stall [14] on the topic of physical abuse. These authors found that parent-child physical abuse, one component of what they termed "adverse familial experiences," was a mediating factor for six sexual risk factors, including having unprotected sex with a non-primary partner and having unprotected sex with a serodiscordant partner. Much more needs to be learned and reported regarding the effects that childhood physical abuse has on HIV risk-taking later in life, and on the effects that other types of childhood maltreatment have on subsequent involvement in risky practices.

Contemporary thinking on the relationship between childhood maltreatment experiences and HIV risk behaviors in adulthood (primarily based on the childhood sexual abuse literature) suggests that the former influences the latter by virtue of their impact upon various aspects of mental health functioning, which in turn is related more closely to risk practices because of its temporal proximity. Rather than conceptualizing the relationship as maltreatment → HIV risk, increasingly, evidence suggests that it is better to conceptualize this relationship as maltreatment → psychological/psychosocial functioning → HIV risk. Studies such as those conducted by Catania and colleagues [8] and Rosario, Schrimshaw, and Hunter [13] have documented just how complicated the effects of childhood maltreatment can be, particularly when trying to link them to adulthood involvement in HIV risk behaviors. Relatively few studies, however, have utilized a structural modeling approach to understand the impact that maltreatment experiences can have on subsequent mental health functioning and risk practices. This is unfortunate, as the complex nature of these interrelationships requires closer study in order to develop truer understandings of the myriad ways in which childhood sexual, physical, and emotional abuse, as well as neglect, may affect adulthood behaviors.

In the present paper, a structural approach is used to develop a better understanding of how childhood maltreatment experiences affect HIV risk involvement in adulthood in a sample of men who use the Internet specifically to find other men with whom they can engage in unprotected sex. Based on previously published studies, the conceptual model depicted in Figure 1 was examined.

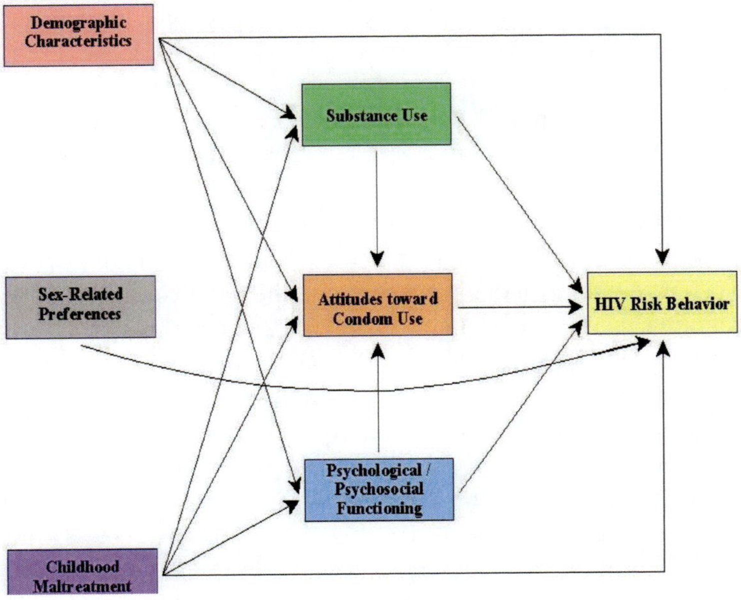

Figure 1. Conceptual Model.

In this exploratory model, childhood maltreatment experiences are hypothesized to have both direct and indirect effects on men's involvement in risky practices. The indirect effects are hypothesized to operate both through the impact of maltreatment on men's psychological/psychosocial functioning, its effects on substance use/abuse, and its impact on their attitudes toward condom use. As the conceptual model shows, childhood maltreatment experiences are one of six types of influences hypothesized to affect men's HIV risk practices. The others are demographic variables (e.g., race/ethnicity, age, HIV serostatus), sex-related behavioral preferences (e.g., self-identification as a sexual "top" versus a "bottom," preferring to have sex that is "wild" or "uninhibited"), substance use/abuse, attitudes toward condom use, and psychological/psychosocial functioning (e.g., depression, self-esteem, impulsivity).

To a great extent, this conceptual model owes its intellectual origins to the notion of syndemic and to Syndemics Theory. "Syndemic" refers to the tendency for multiple epidemics to co-occur and, for the various maladies to interact with one another, with each one worsening the effects of the others [15,16]. Walkup et al [17] noted that health problems may be construed as syndemic when two or more conditions/afflictions are linked in such a manner that they interact synergistically, with each contributing to an excess burden of disease in a particular population. It is noteworthy that their work also addresses the syndemic of HIV, substance abuse, and mental illness. A good example of how conditions may become syndemic is offered by Romero-Daza, Weeks, and Singer [18] in their study of street prostitution. The authors wrote:

> streetwalkers' continuous exposure to violence, both as victims and as witnesses, often leaves them suffering from major emotional trauma. In the absence of adequate support services, women who have been victimized may turn to drug use in an attempt to deal with the harsh realities of their daily lives. In turn, the need for drugs, coupled with a lack of educational and employment opportunities, may lead women into prostitution. Life on the street increases women's risk for physical, emotional, and sexual abuse as well as their risk for HIV/AIDS. Exposure to traumatic experiences deepens the dependence on drugs, completing a vicious cycle of violence, substance abuse, and AIDS risk (pp. 233–234).

Stall and colleagues [19] applied Syndemics Theory to urban MSM's risk for acquiring HIV and focused on the intertwined epidemics of substance abuse, depression, childhood sexual abuse (CSA), and intimate partner violence (IPV). They found that the presence of the co-occurring epidemics increased the likelihood that MSM had engaged in unprotected sex and increased their likelihood of being HIV-positive. A number of authors, particularly during the past few years, have written about syndemics and the Syndemics Theory as they apply to sexual risk taking and the HIV epidemic [16,18,20–22], including specific mention of the applicability of the concept and theory to men who have sex with men [21].

Using the conceptual model shown above, the present study represents an effort to examine the role that childhood maltreatment experiences play in the HIV risk syndemic faced by one population of men who are at particularly great risk of contracting HIV–namely, MSM who use the Internet in search of partners for unprotected sex. The main research questions examined in this exploratory analysis are as follows: (1) How prevalent are experiences with neglect, sexual abuse, physical abuse, and emotional abuse in this population? (2) How, if at all, are these experiences related to men's involvement in HIV risk taking? (3) How, if at all, does childhood maltreatment affect men's psychological/ psychosocial functioning and other factors hypothesized to be related to their HIV risk practices?

Our study

The data reported in this chapter come from The Bareback Project, a National Institute on Drug Abuse-funded study of men who use the Internet specifically to find other men with whom they can engage in unprotected sex. The data were collected between January 2008 and May 2009. A total of 332 men were recruited from 16 different websites. Some of the sites catered exclusively to unprotected sex (e.g., Bareback.com, RawLoads.com) and some of them did not but made it possible for site users to identify which persons were looking for unprotected sex (e.g., Men4SexNow.com, Squirt.org). A nationwide random sample of men was derived, with random selection being based on a combination of the first letter of the person's online username, his race/ethnicity (as listed in his profile), and the day of recruitment. The study design called for an oversampling of men of color, to ensure good representation of racial minority group men in the sample and to facilitate the examination of racial differences in risk taking and risk-related preferences. Recruitment efforts were undertaken seven days a week, during all hours of the day and night, variable from week to week throughout the duration of the project. This was done to maximize the representativeness of the final research sample, in recognition of the fact that different people use the Internet at different times.

Depending upon the website involved, men were approached initially either via instant message or email (much more commonly via email). A brief overview of the study was provided as part of the initial approach and informed consent-related procedures, and all men were given the opportunity to ask questions about the study before deciding whether or not to participate. A website link to the project's online home page was also made available, to provide men with additional information about the project and to help them feel secure about the legitimacy of the research endeavor. Men who were interested in participating were scheduled for an interview, which was conducted as soon after they expressed an interest in taking part in the study as possible, typically within a few days. Interviews were conducted during all hours of the day and night, seven days a week, based on interviewer availability and participants' preferences, to maximize convenience to the participants. All of the study's interviewers were gay or lesbian, to engender credibility with the target population and to enhance participants' comfort during the interviews.

Participation in the study entailed the completion of a one-time, confidential telephone interview covering a wide array of topics. The questionnaire was developed specifically for use in The Bareback Project, with many parts of the interview derived from standardized scales previously used and validated by other researchers. The interview covered such subjects as: degree of "outness," perceived discrimination based on sexual orientation, general health practices, HIV testing history and serostatus, sexual practices (protected and unprotected) with partners met online and offline, risk-related preferences, risk-related hypotheticals, substance use, drug-related problems, Internet usage, psychological and psychosocial functioning, childhood maltreatment experiences, HIV/AIDS knowledge, and some basic demographic information. Interviews lasted an average of 69 minutes (median = 63, s.d. = 20.1, range = 30–210). Men who completed the interview were compensated $35 for their time. Two payment options were offered, one of which allowed men to maintain complete anonymity (PayPal) and one of which required them to provide a name and mailing address to receive payment (check). Prior to implementation in the field, the research protocol was approved by the institutional review boards at Morgan State University (approval number 07/12-0145), where the principal investigator and one of the research assistants were affiliated, and George Mason University (approval number 5659), where the other research assistant was located.

Measures used

The Childhood Trauma Questionnaire [23] was used to examine childhood maltreatment experiences. Six measures, all of which asked men about their experiences prior to the age of 18, were used: sexual abuse (Cronbach's alpha = 0.93), physical abuse (Cronbach's alpha = 0.85), emotional abuse (Cronbach's alpha = 0.89), physical neglect (Cronbach's alpha = 0.71), emotional neglect (Cronbach's alpha = 0.93), and total amount of childhood maltreatment experienced (Cronbach's alpha = 0.94)

The *main outcome measure* (i.e., dependent variable) used in this particular paper indicates the percentage of sex acts that involved the use of protection. It is a continuous measure based on participants' self-reported sexual practices during the 30 days prior to interview.

Numerous measures examining *demographic characteristics* were examined. These included: age (dichotomous, comparing men aged 18–49 years to those aged 50+), race / ethnicity (categorical), relationship status (involved in a marital-type relationship versus not involved), educational attainment (continuous), sexual role identity (top, versatile top, versatile, versatile bottom, bottom), HIV serostatus (positive, negative, unknown), and knowing anyone currently living with AIDS (yes / no).

Four items measuring men's *sex-related preferences* were examined. These were: how rough they preferred their sex to be (continuous), how long they most liked their sexual sessions to last (continuous), how much they liked having sex in public venues (continuous), and how much they liked having sex that was "wild" or "uninhibited" (continuous).

The *substance use / abuse* domain was assessed with three measures: currently a user of illegal drugs (yes / no), number of drug problems experienced (continuous scale measure, Cronbach's alpha = 0.87), and total amount of illegal drug use reported during the preceding 30 days (continuous measure of quantity × frequency of recent use, summed across nine drug types).

Attitudes toward condom use were assessed via a 17-item scale that was found to be highly reliable (Cronbach's alpha = 0.91). Individual items were scored on a five-point Likert scale, and higher scores on the scale corresponded with attitudes that were more conducive of condom use. The scale was derived from the work of Brown [24]. Only items that were relevant to MSM and their sexual practices were used, so that the scale would be applicable to the study population.

Finally, *psychological and psychosocial functioning* were examined. Measures examined were: self-esteem (using the Rosenberg self-esteem scale [25]; Cronbach's alpha = 0.89), depression (using the CES-D [26]); Cronbach's alpha = 0.93), concern about potential sex partners' HIV serostatus (yes / no), and perceived accuracy of HIV serostatus information provided verbally by sex partners (ordinal).

Analysis

The analysis for this research took place in several steps. Initially, bivariate analyses were conducted to examine which of the independent measures were related one-on-one to the dependent measure in question. Whenever the independent variable was dichotomous (e.g., race, sexual orientation), Student's t tests were used. Whenever the independent variable was ordinal with five or more response options or continuous in nature (e.g., extent of sexual abuse, level of self-esteem), simple regression was used to test the bivariate relationships.

Items that were found to be related either significantly ($p<.05$) or marginally ($.15>p>.05$) to the dependent measure in these bivariate analyses were entered into a multivariate equation, and then removed in stepwise fashion until a best fit model containing only statistically-significant measures remained. This approach was used for the main outcome measure (i.e., percentage of protected sex) and for each of the relevant endogenous measures (e.g., condom-related attitudes, level of self-esteem).

As a final analytical step, the relationships depicted in Figure 2 (which portray the results of the analyses just described) were subjected to a structural equation analysis to determine whether the way the relationships depicted there are an appropriate and effective representation of the study data. SAS's PROC CALIS procedure was used to assess the overall fit of the model to the data. When conducting a structural equation analysis, several specific characteristics are examined and sought: (1) a goodness-of-fit index as close to 1.00 as possible, but no less than 0.90, (2) a Bentler-Bonett normed fit index value as close to 1.00 as possible, but no less than 0.90, (3) an overall chi-square value for the model that is statistically nonsignificant, preferably as far from attaining statistical significance as possible, and (4) a root mean square error approximation value as close to 0.00 as possible, but no greater than 0.05. If these conditions are met, then the structural relationships depicted are considered to indicate a good fit with the data.

Throughout all of the analyses, results are reported as statistically significant whenever $p<.05$.

Our findings

In total, 332 men participated in the study. They ranged in age from 18 to 72 (mean = 43.7, s.d. = 11.2, median = 43.2). Racially, the sample is a fairly close approximation of the American population, with 74.1% being Caucasian, 9.0% each being African American and Latino, 5.1% self-identifying as biracial or multiracial, 2.4% being Asian, and 0.3% being Native American. The large majority of the men (89.5%) considered themselves to be gay; 10.2% said they were bisexual; and 0.3% self-identified as "curious." On balance, men participating in The Bareback Project were fairly well-educated. About 1 man in 7 (14.5%) had completed no more than high school; 34.3% had some college experience without earning a college degree; 28.9% had a bachelor's degree; and 22.3% were educated beyond the bachelor's level. Slightly more than one-half of the men (59.0%) reported being HIV-positive; most of the rest (38.6%) were HIV-negative; and some men (2.4%) did not know about their current HIV serostatus.

Maltreatment experiences during men's formative years were quite prevalent in this study population. It should be noted that the following figures provide conservative, low-end prevalence figures because responses of "rarely" to the component items are not being counted as affirmative in the reporting of these "yes/no" childhood maltreatment summary measures. (Please note that, in computing the scale measures used in the remainder of the analyses for this paper, raw data values are summed, including the appropriate differentiations of values for the "never" and "rarely" responses.) Nearly two-thirds of the men (61.7%) gave answers indicating that they had been abused emotionally. More than one-half (51.1%) had been abused physically at least sometimes. More than one-quarter (25.5%) reported having been sexually abused "sometimes," "often," or "very often" before the age of 18. More than one-half of the men (52.0%) had been victims of emotional neglect and more than one-third (34.4%) had been physically neglected during their formative years. Overall, 80.6% of the men reported at least one of these forms of maltreatment during their childhood and/or adolescent years.

Childhood maltreatment and HIV risk practices

Contrary to our initial research hypothesis, childhood maltreatment experiences were not found to be related to men's involvement in risky sex. This was true for sexual abuse (p=.534), physical abuse (p=.568), emotional abuse (p=.352), emotional neglect (p=.433), physical neglect (p=.852), and the total amount of maltreatment (p=.666) alike.

Childhood maltreatment and attitudes toward condom use

In the bivariate analyses, three of the six childhood maltreatment measures were found to be associated with men's attitudes toward condom use. In each instance, the more maltreatment that men experienced during their formative years, the worse their attitudes toward using condoms tended to be in adulthood. This was true with regard to emotional abuse ($F_{1,327df}$=5.80, p=.017), emotional neglect ($F_{1,327df}$=8.85, p=.003), and the total amount of maltreatment experienced ($F_{1,327df}$=4.88, p=.028).

When these measures were added to the multivariate equation, however, none of them was retained as a statistically significant contributor once the effects of other measures were taken into account. As Figure 2 demonstrates, the effects of childhood maltreatment on attitudes toward condom use were secondary to those of seven other measures. Condom-related attitudes were reported by men who: were African American (p=.008), had a lower amount of education (p=.009), cared about their sex partners' HIV serostatus (p=.004), had a lesser preference for engaging in "wild or uninhibited" sex (p<.001), had fewer problems resulting from substance abuse (p=.009), perceived their sex partners to be less truthful about their HIV serostatus when discussing the subject with them (p=.004), and those who had a higher self-esteem (p=.002).

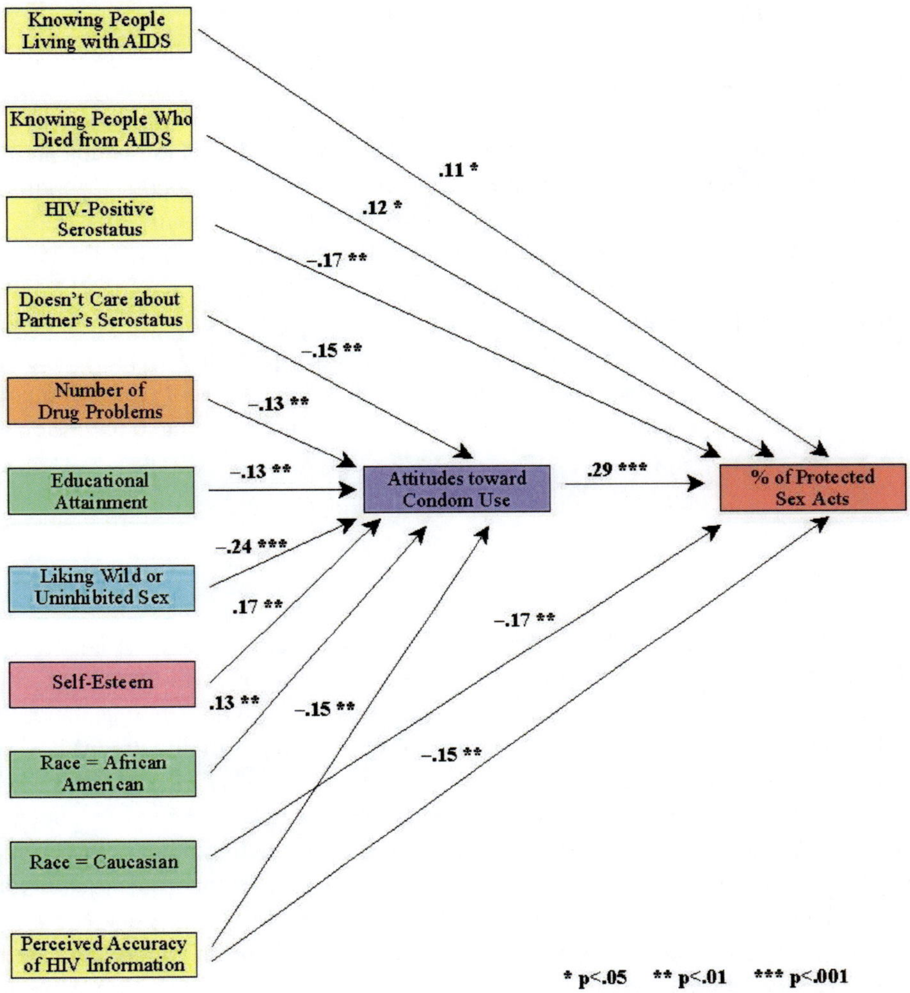

Figure 2. Condom-Related Attitudes and Protected Sex.

Childhood maltreatment and self-esteem

In the bivariate analyses, four of the six childhood maltreatment measures were found to be predictive of men's levels of self-esteem. In all four of these instances, greater maltreatment was associated with lower self-esteem. This was true with regard to emotional abuse ($F_{1,327df}$=24.69, p<.001), emotional neglect ($F_{1,327df}$=36.34, p<.001), physical neglect ($F_{1,327df}$=29.69, p<.001), and the total amount of maltreatment experienced ($F_{1,327df}$=22.70, p<.001).

As Figure 2 depicts, when these items were entered into the multivariate equation, one of them–emotional neglect–was found to contribute uniquely and significantly to the overall prediction of men's levels of self-esteem (p<.001). Also predictive of lower levels of self-esteem were race (specifically, not being African American, p=.008), lower educational attainment (p=.009), being under the age of 50 (p=.047), and being overweight (p=.027).

Testing the structural equation model shown in figure 2

As a final analytical step, the results of the multivariate analyses were subjected to a structural equation analysis, to examine the totality of the relationships portrayed in Figure 2. This analysis provided strong confirmatory support for the way that the relationships are depicted there. When conducting structural equation analysis, we want to obtain a goodness-of-fit index that is greater than 0.900. For this equation, the coefficient was 0.987. When conducting structural equation analysis, we want a Bentler-Bonett normed fit index that is greater than 0.900. For this equation, the coefficient was 0.946. In this type of analysis, we strive for an overall chi-square value for the model that is statistically nonsignificant, preferably as far from attaining statistical significance as possible. Here, it was p=.213. Finally, using structural equation modeling, we strive for a root mean square error approximation value as close to 0.00 as possible, but no greater than 0.050. Here, it was 0.028.

Discussion

One of this study's main hypotheses was that childhood maltreatment would be related to men's involvement in HIV risk practices. To our surprise, however, in this study, childhood maltreatment had no direct effect on men's HIV risk taking. This finding stands in clear contrast to most of the published literature that shows childhood maltreatment is associated with greater HIV risk taking. [5,7–14]

This is not to say, however, that childhood maltreatment is irrelevant to understanding risk in this population. As Figure 2 demonstrates, childhood maltreatment *is* important in the overall prediction of men's HIV risk behavior, but its effect was found to be indirect rather than direct. The relationship of childhood maltreatment to HIV risk behavior appears to operate in the following manner: Men's experiences of childhood maltreatment lowers their self-esteem. Lower self-esteem, in turn, alters their attitudes towards using condoms in a negative manner and that, in turn, ultimately increases their likelihood of engaging in unprotected sex. Thus, in the present study population, childhood maltreatment experiences appeared to be operating "in the background" when it comes to their influence on HIV risk taking in adulthood.

In recent years, there has been increasing support in the scientific community for the notion that childhood maltreatment experiences are complex in terms of how they affect people later in life. Although many studies [5,7–13] have suggested that childhood maltreatment has a direct effect upon risk taking, increasingly, evidence suggests that maltreatment operates through a variety of "intermediary" or "mediating" mechanisms when having long-term effects on people. Studies such as those conducted by Catania and colleagues [8] and Rosario, Schrimshaw, and Hunter [13] have documented just how complicated the effects of childhood maltreatment can be, particularly when trying to link them to adulthood involvement in HIV risk behaviors. Our findings support the main contentions of these researchers, and suggest that future research in this area would be well-advised to examine exactly how it is that childhood maltreatment leads to greater risk taking later in life. In particular, we believe that research focusing on the psychological and psychosocial effects of being maltreated, and how exactly it is that these psychological/ psychosocial effects are related to subsequent risk behavior taking, would be beneficial and informative to the scientific community.

In addition to the preceding, we would also like to point out that, in this study, the single most useful, or applicable, measure of childhood maltreatment was emotional neglect. This stands in contrast to most of the previously-published studies, which generally have focused specifically on sexual abuse. In the analyses conducted in conjunction with the present research, the total amount of childhood maltreatment experienced was related to men's levels of self-esteem; but the extent to which they had been victims of emotional neglect during their formative years was related to their levels of self-esteem more closely. When one considers the types of items that comprised the emotional neglect subscale (e.g., "You felt loved" or "Someone in your family helped you feel important or special"), it makes perfect sense that men who had been emotionally neglected during their formative years would have lower self-esteem as adults. They felt isolated as a child/adolescent and did not feel that they had the love and support that society says ought to be there for them. Additionally, it stands to reason that feelings of emotional abandonment and familial betrayal—betrayal of what society tells them they should expect from members of their immediate family—will have a negative impact on a man's self-esteem. A person's self-esteem and sense of self—who he is in the world—are formed when he is young. If he grows up with a good sense of self, then that is likely to remain with him throughout his lifetime. Alternatively, if he suffered from emotional neglect and does not have a good opinion of himself, he is likely to suffer long-term consequences if he does not receive help and counseling to increase his self-esteem.

In conclusion, this study found that childhood maltreatment is important in predicting HIV risk taking in this population of high risk MSM, but not in a manner that has been shown by most other published studies. In this study, emotional neglect was the single most influential measurement of childhood maltreatment that affected HIV risk behavior. It did so by lowering men's levels of self-esteem, which in turn altered their feelings about using condoms in a negative manner, which in turn led them to be less likely to practice protected sex. Future research should attempt to replicate these findings in other populations of MSM to see if they are replicable. If so, this would indicate that HIV prevention interventionists need to address the lasting negative sequelae associated with emotional neglect in childhood—mainly low self-esteem—to interrupt the pathway between childhood emotional neglect and engaging in unprotected sex.

Acknowledgments

This research was supported by a grant from the National Institute on Drug Abuse (R24-DA019805). The authors would like to acknowledge, with gratitude, the significant contribution made to the study's data collection, data entry, and data cleaning efforts by Thomas P. Lambing.

References

[1] McCauley J, Kern DE, Kolodner K, Dill L, Schroder AF, DeChant HK, et al. Clinical characteristics of women with a history of childhood abuse: Unhealed wounds. *JAMA* 1997;277:1362-8.

[2] Bensley LS, VanEenwyk J, Simmons KW. Self-reported childhood sexual and physical abuse and adult HIV-risk behaviors and heavy drinking. *Am. J. Prev. Med.* 2000;18:151-8.

[3] Mimiaga MJ, Noonan E, Donnell D, Safren SA, Koenen KC, Gortmaker S, et al. Childhood sexual abuse is highly associated with HIV risk-taking behavior and infection among MSM in the EXPLORE Study. *J. Acquir Immune Defic. Syndr.* 2009;51:340-8.

[4] Smith HA, Markovic N, Danielson ME, Matthews A, Youk A, Talbott EO, Larkby C, Hughes T. Sexual abuse, sexual orientation, and obesity in women. *J. Womens Health* 2010;19:1525-32.

[5] Dorais M. Hazardous journey of intimacy: HIV transmission risk behaviors of young men who are victims of past sexual abuses and who have sexual relations with men. *J. Homosex,* 2004;48:103-24.

[6] Schraufnagela TJ, Davis KS, George WH, Norris J. Childhood sexual abuse in males and subsequent risky sexual behavior: A potential alcohol-use pathway. *Child Abuse Negl.* 2010;34:369-78.

[7] Fields SD, Malebranche D, Feist-Price S. Childhood sexual abuse in black men who have sex with men: Results from three qualitative studies. *Cultur Divers Ethnic Minor Psychol.,* 2008;14:385-90.

[8] Catania JA, Paul J, Osmond D, Folkman S, Pollack L, Canchola J, Chang J, Nellands T. Mediators of childhood sexual abuse and high-risk sex among men-who-have-sex-with-men. *Child Abuse Negl.* 2008;32:925-40.

[9] O'Leary A, Purcell D, Remien RH, Gomez C. Childhood sexual abuse and sexual transmission risk behaviour among HIV-positive men who have sex with men. *AIDS Care* 2003:15:17-26.

[10] Brennan DJ, Hellerstedt WL, Ross MW, Welles SL. History of childhood sexual abuse and HIV risk behaviors in homosexual and bisexual men. *Am. J. Public Health* 2007;97:1107-12.

[11] Gore-Felton C, Kalichman SC, Brondino MJ, Benotsch EG, Cage M, DiFonzo K. Childhood sexual abuse and HIV risk among men who have sex with men: Initial test of a conceptual model. *J. Fam. Violence* 2006;21:263-70.

[12] Saewyc E, Skay C, Richens K, Reis E, Poon C, Murphy A. Sexual orientation, sexual abuse, and HIV-risk behaviors among adolescents in the Pacific Northwest. *Am. J. Public Health* 2006;96:1104-10.

[13] Rosario M, Schrimshaw EW, Hunter J. A model of sexual risk behaviors among young gay and bisexual men: Longitudinal associations of mental health, substance abuse, sexual abuse, and the coming-out process. *AIDS Educ. Prev.* 2006;18:444-60.

[14] Paul JP, Catania J, Pollack L, Stall R. Understanding childhood sexual abuse as a predictor of sexual risk-taking among men who have sex with men: The Urban Men's Health Study. *Child Abuse Negl.* 2001;25:557-84.

[15] Singer M. Introduction to syndemics: A systems approach to public and community health. San Francisco, CA: Jossey-Bass, 2009.

[16] Singer MC, Erickson PI, Badiane L, Diaz R, Ortiz D, Abraham T, Nicolaysen AM. Syndemics, sex and the city: Understanding sexually transmitted diseases in social and cultural context. *Soc. Sci. Med.,* 2006;63:2010-21.

[17] Walkup J, Blank MB, Gonzales JS, Safren S, Schwartz R, Brown L, et al. The impact of mental health and substance abuse factors on HIV prevention and treatment. *J. Acquir Immune Defic. Syndr.* 2008; 47:s15-9.

[18] Romero-Daza N, Weeks M, Singer M. "Nobody gives a damn if I live or die": Violence, drugs, and street-level prostitution in inner-city Hartford, Connecticut. *Med. Anthropol* 2003;22:233-59.

[19] Stall R, Mills T, Williamson J, Hart T. Association of co-occurring psychosocial health problems and increased vulnerability to HIV/AIDS among urban men who have sex with men. *Am. J. Public Health* 2003;93:939-42.

[20] Gielen AC, Ghandour RM, Burke JG, Mahoney P, McDonnell KA, O'Campo P. HIV/AIDS and intimate partner violence: Intersecting women's health issues in the United States. *Trauma Violence Abuse,* 2007;8:178-98.

[21] Mustanski B, Garofalo R, Herrick A, Donenberg G. Psychosocial health problems increase risk for HIV among urban young men who have sex with men: Preliminary evidence of a syndemic in need of attention. *Ann. Behav. Med.* 2007;34:37-45.

[22] Senn TE, Carey MP, Vanable PA. The intersection of violence, substance use, depression, and STDs: Testing of a syndemic pattern among patients attending an urban STD clinic. *J. Natl. Med. Assoc.* 2010;102:614-20.

[23] Bernstein DP, Fink L. *Childhood Trauma Questionnaire: A retrospective self-report manual.* San Antonio, TX: Psychological Corporation, 1998.

[24] Brown IS. Development of a scale to measure attitude toward the condom as a method of birth control. *J. Sex Res.* 1984;20:255-63.

[25] Rosenberg M. *Society and the adolescent self-image.* Princeton, NJ: Princeton University Press, 1965.

[26] Radloff LS. The CES-D scale: A self-report depression scale for research in the general population. *Appl. Psychol. Meas* 1977;1:385-401.

In: Human Immunodeficiency Virus …
Editors: Hugh Klein and Joav Merrick

ISBN: 978-1-62081-293-8

Chapter IV

Understanding the agreements and behaviors of men who have sex with men who are dating or married to women: Unexpected implications for a universal HIV/STI testing protocol

Jason W. Mitchell,[1] David A. Moskowitz[2,*] and David W. Seal[3]

[1]Center for AIDS Intervention Research, Department of Psychiatry and Behavioral Medicine, Medical College of Wisconsin, Milwaukee, Wisconsin, US

[2]Department of Communication, University of Texas at San Antonio, Texas US

[3]Department of Global Community Health and Behavioral Sciences, School of Public Health and Tropical Medicine, Tulane University, New Orleans, Louisianna, US

Abstract

Men with a female partner who also have sex with men (MSMW) have been identified as a bridge population for possible HIV transmission to heterosexual women. Social science research that examines how relational and social aspects of MSMW partnered with women is needed to better understand the possible mechanisms that may contribute to HIV/STI risk among MSMW, their female relationship partners, and secondary male sex partners. Our study assessed whether self-reported accounts of sexual agreements and relationship behaviors of MSMW with a current female partner corresponded to their sexual risk behaviors with secondary male sex partners. A cross-sectional study design was used to collect anonymous data from a convenience sample of 145 MSMW who had a current female partner and also sought to engage in sex with men. The data indicated that the majority of MSMW engaged in oral and/or anal sex with another male without their female partner knowing. Of men reporting strictly monogamous heterosexual relationships, only 14.5% reported actually only having sex with their female relational

* Correspondence: David A Moskowitz, PhD, University of Texas at San Antonio, One UTSA Circle, Dept. of Communication, San Antonio, Texas 78249 United States. E-mail: david.moskowitz@utsa.edu.

partner. The men's average last tests for HIV and STIs were 87.5 and 181.9 months prior, respectively; and most men self-reported low condom use during oral sex and inconsistent condom use during anal intercourse. Universal HIV/STI testing is urgently needed to improve testing rates among MSMW who are unlikely to admit risk-behaviors. Additionally, tailored HIV prevention strategies such as couples-based sexuality and HIV/STI counseling may be beneficial for MSMW.

Introduction

Although men who have sex with men (MSM) are estimated to represent two to five percent of the population, more than half of all new HIV infections each year are among MSM in the United States [1]. The primary sexual risk factor for HIV transmission between MSM is unprotected anal intercourse (UAI) [2]; yet, not all MSM solely engage in male-to-male sex. Additionally, heterosexual women account for almost one-third of individuals infected by HIV and are more susceptible to HIV infection through unprotected vaginal intercourse than are heterosexual men [3,4]. Hypothetically, men who have UAI with other men and unprotected vaginal intercourse or UAI with women may increase new HIV infections among heterosexual women, and help sustain the disproportionate impact of HIV/AIDS among MSM. Prior research has supported this notion that men who engage in sexual risk behaviors with both men and women (MSMW) may serve as a bridge population for HIV transmission [5-11]. Because many of these specific men are partnered, social aspects that help to create and maintain their relationships ultimately might be the key predictors of protective or, alternatively, risky sexual health behaviors.

In response to how HIV may be transmitted through bridge populations, a growing body of research has emerged to examine the social and relational characteristics and dynamics of men in concurrent sexual partnerships. Research with MSMW, either labeled as non-gay identified or behaviorally bisexual men, has examined sexual risk behaviors to determine the likelihood of HIV and STI transmission to female sex partners. Published data on MSMW indicated several individual characteristics that are associated with an increase in sexual risk behaviors, including: 1) having sex with both men and women, 2) a non-gay identity, and 3) concealment of same-sex behavior from female partners [9, 12-19]. Other research has examined correlates and reasons for why MSMW use condoms and test for HIV less frequently [19-22].

However, gaps in the HIV prevention literature, which deal specifically with the social/relational aspects of MSMW, remain understudied. Few studies have collected and described self-reported sexual risk behavior and relationship data, including agreements of MSMW who actively placed advertisements on the Internet (i.e., www.craigslist.org) for same-sex encounters. Moreover, little is known about the association between self-reported data on relationship behaviors and relationship agreements among MSMW with their female partners and the sexual risk behaviors in which MSMW engage with male secondary sex partners. Research that examines the intersection of these important social aspects (specifically, the concordance/discordance of sexual behaviors and agreements with relationship partners among MSMW) is needed in order to design suitable HIV/STI prevention interventions.

The present study sought to assess whether self-reported accounts of sexual agreements and relationship behaviors of MSMW with a steady female partner corresponded to their sexual risk behaviors with secondary male sex partners. The overall aim of the present research was to expand our understanding of the contributing factors, including relationship agreements, to HIV and STI risk transmission among MSMW, their female relationship partners, and any secondary male sex partners they may have. Specifically, this study has three objectives: 1) to describe the distribution of relationship types, agreements, and self-reported sexual behaviors (including condom use) among female partnered MSMW who actively sought out and engaged in sexual behaviors with men; 2) to examine the degree to which agreements match with behaviors among MSMW; and 3) to assess the differences and similarities of self-reported relationship agreements and sexual risk behaviors among the sample.

Our study

Men, regardless of sexual identity, who placed an advertisement to engage in sex with other men on each Craigslist.org mirror website where English was the primary language, were invited to take a brief online survey. Various cities and locations throughout the US have a Craigslist.org website assigned to their respective location (i.e., a mirror website). Each Craigslist.org location in the U.S. was used to recruit for the present study. The first one hundred men's sexual advertisements at each of the Craigslist websites were selected to receive a block message that informed them of our research study. A link embedded in the email took them directly to the anonymous survey. The first page contained a consent form. Participants could not advance to the actual survey without first consenting. Participants were not compensated for their time. After excluding men who did not complete all of the necessary information to answer our research questions (n = 193) and those who were either single (n = 328) or partnered with a male (n = 157), a sample of 145 men was left for our analysis. We purposely excluded men who reported being single and those who were partnered with a male due to our research interest in the dynamics of concurrent sexual partnerships among female-partnered men who were seeking male-to-male sexual behaviors. Data from 145 men with current female partners who also sought sex with males were used to examine our objectives.

Measures used

Basic demographic data were elicited: sexual identity, age, city size, race/ethnicity, income, education, self-reported HIV serostatus, and number of months since last reported HIV and STI test. Participants were asked to categorize their sexual identity as 'heterosexual', 'homosexual', 'bisexual', or 'will not label'. City size options included, '< 10,000 persons', '10,000 – 50,000 persons', '51,000 – 100,000 persons', '101,000 – 500,000 persons', '501,000 – 1 million persons', and 'over 1 million persons'. Education level was obtained through the following categories: 'finished some high school', 'graduated high school', 'graduated high school and finished some college, 'graduated college, 'graduated college and finished some graduate work', and 'received a graduate degree'.

Relationship type and length

To assess relationship type, we asked participants to check one of the following categories: 1) 'I'm single, not involved in a relationship'; 2) 'I'm in a non-cohabitating relationship with a woman (you're not living together)'; 3) 'I'm in a cohabitating relationship with a woman (you're living together)'; and 4) 'I'm legally married to, or have a civil union with, a woman'. As previously mentioned, men who chose category one (i.e., who were single) were excluded from our analyses, as were men who admitted to dating or being involved with another man. The men indicated the length of their current relationship in months.

Relationship agreement

To capture the diversity in relationship agreements that participants may have had with their female partners, we asked which category best described the sort of agreement they had with their current main partner. These were: 1) 'implicitly monogamous (without talking about it, you and your partner just know you are monogamous)'; 2) 'explicitly monogamous (you and your partner have actually discussed that you both will be monogamous)'; 3) 'non-monogamous, but you tell your main partner when you have fooled around with other individuals'; 4) 'non-monogamous, but you do not tell your main partner when you have fooled around with other individuals'; and 5) 'non-monogamous, but only when both you and your partner fool around with another person together (you only have threesomes with you, your partner, and a third person)'.

Male-to-male sexual behaviors with or without female partner

Participants were asked to select the statement that best described the sort of same-sex sexual behaviors enacted while being in their current relationship. These statements were: 1) 'I have only ever fooled around or had sex with my partner'; 2) 'I have fooled around with other men WITHOUT my partner being there and have had oral intercourse but HAVE NOT had anal intercourse'; 3) 'I have fooled around with other men WITHOUT my partner being there and have had oral AND anal intercourse'; 4) 'I have fooled around with other men WITH my partner being there and have had oral intercourse but HAVE NOT had anal intercourse'; and 5) 'I have fooled around with other men WITH my partner being there and have had oral and anal intercourse'. Because not all sexual behaviors that men engage in were addressed with this measure, one potential limitation is the assessment of men who had anal sex, but not oral sex, with or without the female partner being there.

Relationship partner's awareness of male-to-male sexual behaviors

Married men (who comprised the overwhelming majority of the sample) were asked whether their female partners were aware of their same-sex behaviors. Participants responded to the following statement, "I am currently married to my wife, and she DOES know about my hooking up with other men", by selecting either 'yes' or 'no'.

Number of male sex partners

Men were asked to indicate the number of male sex partners they had accrued over the previous 12 months for oral intercourse. An additional question was asked to obtain data on how many male sex partners the men had for anal intercourse in the previous 12 months.

Condom use

Men were asked the following two questions, "In the past 12 months, what percent of the time did you use condoms during oral intercourse when having sex with men?" and "In the past 12 months, what percent of the time did you use condoms during anal intercourse when having sex with men?" For each measure regarding condom use, participants were given eight possible responses: 1) 'I never had this sort of sexual partner'; 2) 'I never used a condom'; 3) 'I practically never used a condom'; 4) 'I rarely used a condom'; 5) 'I sometimes used a condom'; 6) 'I usually used a condom'; 7) 'I practically always used a condom'; and 8) 'I always used a condom'. These categories were collapsed into 'always', 'sometimes', and 'never' wears a condom for both oral and anal sex behaviors (where "sometimes" was comprised of individuals who selected answers three through seven). MSMW selecting, "I never had this sort of partner," were excluded from the individual analyses.

Analysis

Stata/SE Version 11 (StataCorp LP, College Station, TX) for Mac was used to conduct all analyses. Descriptive statistics were calculated to describe the study sample's demographics, relationship characteristics, sexual behaviors, and lack of condom use for oral and anal sex with males. Pearson's chi-square test was then used to assess the degree to which participants' relationship agreements and relationship sexual behaviors were concordant or discordant. The independent t-test was used to assess differences among participants' self-reported relationship agreements, relationship sexual behaviors, and agreement-behavior discordance for their last reported HIV and STI tests, and condom use.

Missing data were present in the measures for relationship duration, sexual risk behaviors with males, and condom use with males. Most notably, forty percent of the men did not report how long they have been in their current relationship with their female partner. It remains unclear as to why so many men did not report how long they have been in their current relationship with their female partner. Future research must take into account this limitation and its possible, significant bias. Missing data on other measures were minimal and are noted when the results are presented.

What did we find?

Demographic and relationship characteristics for the sample are presented in table 1. The mean age for participants was 44.7 years (SD = 12.1); men as young as 19 and as old as 79 years participated in the study. The majority of the sample self-identified as: White (88%); bisexual (75%); and married to their female partner (79%). Most men also had completed some college or attained a bachelor's degree (66.7%); earned at least $50,000 (63.9%); and lived in locales with a population of 100,000 persons or less (51.4%).

Table 1. Demographic and relationship characteristics of 145 MSMW study participants

Characteristic	% (N)
Race	
White	88.3% (128)
Latino	6.2% (9)
African American	1.4% (2)
Indian	1.4% (2)
Other	2.7% (4)
Sexuality	
Heterosexual	12.4% (18)
Homosexual	6.2% (9)
Bisexual	73.8% (107)
Chose no label	7.6% (11)
Self-reported HIV serostatus	
Negative	93.8% (136)
Positive	1.4% (2)
Unknown	4.8% (7)
Relationship status	
Dating a female partner	10.3% (15)
Living with female partner	11.0% (16)
Married to a female partner	78.6% (114)
Relationship agreement	
Implicit monogamy	22.1% (32)
Explicit monogamy	15.9% (23)
Non-monogamous: Disclose when unfaithful	8.3% (12)
Non-monogamous: Does not disclose when unfaithful	51.0% (74)
Non-monogamous: Threesomes or partner knows	2.8% (4)
Self-reported sexual behaviors with or without female partner	
Only had sex with female partner	5.5% (8)
Had oral and/or anal sex; female partner not present	89.0% (129)

Characteristic	% (N)
Had oral and/or anal sex; female partner present	5.5% (8)
Female partner knows about sexual behaviors with men[c]	10.3% (15)
	Mean (SD), [Range]
Age (years)	44.7 (12.1), [19 – 79]
Relationship duration (months)[a]	211.3 (142.9), [9 – 562]
Last HIV test (months)[b]	87.5 (125.0), [0 – 289]
Last STD test (months)[b]	181.9 (225.1), [0 – 481]

[a] Approximately 40% of the sample did not respond to this measure (i.e., 58 missing cases).
[b] Twenty-four men did not respond to these measures.
[c] Applicable to married men only.

Table 2. MSMW self-reported sexual risk behaviors and condom use with male secondary sex partners

Sexual risk behavior[a]	*Mean* (SD), [Range]
Oral sex with male	15.4 (26.8), [0 – 200]
Anal sex with male	5.1 (14.5), [0 – 100]
Condom use: Never[b]	% (*n*)
Oral sex with male	67.3% (74)
Anal sex with male	13.7% (10)
Condom use: Sometimes[b]	% (*n*)
Oral sex with male	28.2% (31)
Anal sex with male	58.9% (43)
Condom use: Always[b]	% (*n*)
Oral sex with male	4.5% (5)
Anal sex with male	27.4% (20)

[a] Minimal missing data occurred for MSMW's self-reported sexual risk behaviors with males (9 cases). Not all MSMW had oral and/or anal sex with another male. Thirteen MSMW self-reported no oral sex with a male. Sixty-three MSMW self-reported no anal sex with a male.
[b] Missing data occurred for MSMW's self-reported condom use with males (24 cases). Regarding condom use with males, eleven MSMW self-reported no oral sex with a male. Forty-eight MSMW self-reported no anal sex with a male.

The proportion of men from small- to medium-sized towns was due to our sampling technique of selecting craigslist.org mirror-sites for cities and towns that varied in population size (e.g., NYC.craigslist.org, Asheville.craigslist.org, Anchorage.craigslist.org, etc.).

Findings

Approximately one-half of the men indicated that their current relationship was non-monogamous without disclosing to their current female partner when they were unfaithful. Furthermore, 89% of the men self-reported that they had oral and/or anal sex with another male without their female partner being present. However, 10% of men did report that their female partners knew about their sexual behaviors with men.

Table 1 shows the distribution of relationship types, agreements, and extra-relationship behaviors. In terms of how well the agreements correspond to actual and allowed behaviors, there were key differences in concordance and discordance (χ^2 (6, 137) = 58.27, ϕ^2 = .40, p < .001). Of men reporting strictly monogamous heterosexual relationships, only 14.5% actually reported having sex with only their relational partner. Most monogamous men (80.0%) reported having sex with others without their partner present. A few monogamous men (5.5%) reported have sex with others with their partner present. Although these men reported being in a strictly monogamous heterosexual relationship, the data indicated that, in reality, sex was occurring outside of their relationship and without their partner being there. Of men reporting non-monogamous relationships in which they disclose extra-relationship sexual encounters, 0.0% reported only having sex with their relational partner, 83.3% reported sex without their partner present, and 16.7% reported sex with their partner present. Of men reporting non-monogamous relationships in which they do not disclose extra-relationship sexual encounters, 0.0% reported only having sex with their relational partner, 100.0% reported sex without their partner present, and 0.0% reported sex with their partner present. Finally, of men only engaging in threesomes, 0.0% reported only having sex with their relational partner, 25.0% reported sex without their partner present, and 75.0% reported sex with their partner present.

Table 2 provides data on participants' self-reported sexual risk behaviors and condom use with male partners. Over the previous 12 months, men reported an average of 15 male partners for oral sex and 5 male partners for anal sex. Not all men with a female partner reported having oral or anal sex with another male in the previous 12 months. Of the men who did (n = 121, 83%), some had oral and/or anal sex with another male without using a condom. About two-thirds of those reporting never used a condom for oral sex with a male. Approximately 14% of MSMW 'never' used a condom for anal sex with a male; 59% reported 'sometimes' or inconsistently used condoms for anal sex with a male; and 27% of men stated that they 'always' used a condom for anal sex with another male. Most surprisingly, the average times since last HIV and STI test were approximately 7 years, 4 months and 15 years, 2 months, respectively. That is, considering the number of partners accrued each year and the lapse in HIV/STI testing, the average MSMW in our sample could not possibly be certain of his HIV/STI status.

No significant statistical differences were found between men's reported last HIV and STI test by relationship agreement or relationship sexual behaviors. Further, neither number of oral/anal sex partners nor condom use statistically differed by participants' relationship agreement type, relationship sexual behaviors, or agreement-behavior discordance.

Discussion

Behavioral and structural HIV and STI prevention interventions that focus on improving the HIV/STI testing behaviors of MSMW, sexual health, and related communication within relationships are urgently needed for behaviorally bisexual individuals, including MSMW who currently have a female relationship partner. Findings from the present study highlight the disconnect that exists between men's reported relationship agreements, relationship behaviors regarding sex with or without their current female partner, and sexual risk behaviors (e.g., inconsistent condom use) in which they engage with secondary male sex partners. Simply put, most MSMW in this sample were not talking with their female relationship partners about their engagements in sexual behaviors with men, were using condoms inconsistently during anal intercourse, and were not getting HIV/STI tested. In many instances, the men were actively breaking their expressed monogamous agreements.

The lack of HIV and STI testing and inconsistent rates of condom use during oral and anal intercourse with male partners is of concern. These trends highlight the potential for the unknowing transmission of STIs and HIV to female relationship partners of MSMW. For example, the average time since their last HIV/STI test was more than seven years. Given this lapse, it is likely that the men might have contracted one of the less manifest STIs (e.g., HIV, HPV, Chlamydia) and potentially, may have transmitted such infections to partners. To speculate on these low testing rates: MSMW may not consider themselves at risk for STIs and HIV because they do not consider themselves "gay." Generally, there may be a disconnect between the behaviors practiced by MSMW and their perceptions of the risks associated with these behaviors—a disconnect that MSM and gay men may not make. Our findings of lapsed HIV and STI testing and infrequent use of condoms among MSMW further contribute and support what previous research has found with bisexual men in the U.S. [19, 20, 22]. Our results are also quantitative, represent MSMW throughout the U.S., and further highlight the lack of disclosure about male-to-male sexual behaviors to their steady female partners.

The present research provides strong evidence for the need for universal STI and HIV testing by healthcare providers. Simply, all men and women should be tested. The low testing rates coupled with the men not mentioning their male-to-male sexual behaviors to their female partners, is worrisome for preventing STIs and transmission of HIV. Hypothetically, some women partnered to these men might not recognize their inadvertent risk for STIs and HIV and the need to get tested. They unknowingly may be providing their primary healthcare provider or gynecologist with misinformation about their relationship and related sexual behaviors. Additionally, a similar trend might be occurring when MSMW visit their primary care physicians. Stigma, shame, guilt, or perceptions of being judged may act as obstacles towards truthful and full patient-provider communication. To circumvent these two possible scenarios, universal testing, regardless of an admission of risk, is necessary. In addition to universal testing, programs that encourage both partners within the couple to communicate about their relationship and sexual health are urgently needed, essential, and necessary for preventing HIV and other STIs.

Condom use was not particularly consistent during anal intercourse, with seven out of ten men reporting inconsistent or absent condom use. This trend did not vary between different groups of MSMW, or between those with concordant or discordant relationship agreements and behaviors. While the number of anal male partners was relatively low compared with number of oral intercourse partners (about 10 fewer per year on average), the risk of infection of STIs and HIV significantly increases for unprotected anal intercourse [23]. It only takes one unprotected experience to transmit disease. Ultimately, many of these men are making sexual health decisions for their female partners, who may be operating under the assumption of monogamy. Tailored intervention programs that help MSMW come out of the proverbial closet and address their same-sex sexual encounters with their partners are needed. However, this is no small task. Shame, alienation, guilt, and the likelihood of divorce all may act as disincentives to truthful communication. MSMW alternatively may prefer to engage in sex with other men without disclosing such acts to their steady female partners because of the thrill that they experience. In the final analysis, and considering the average man in this sample was in his mid-forties, coming to terms with an unconventional sexuality may be too difficult and disruptive for MSMW. A structural intervention (e.g., a universal HIV/STI testing protocol) may be an optimal way to circumvent the difficulties of interpersonal disclosures. Such a protocol would allow healthcare providers to identify men who may have contracted diseases before they transmit them to their female partner or secondary male partners.

Limitations

Despite these key findings, our research did have limitations related to missing data (i.e. overall condom use and relationship duration), lack of data to conclude the degree to which the MSMW also were sexually active specifically with their current female partner, recall bias, and the inability to determine causality or temporal associations among the various relationship factors and sexual risk behaviors. Our research also did not collect data on every possible sexual encounter of MSMW's male-to-male sexual behaviors with or without their female partner (i.e., men who had anal sex, but not oral sex, with or without the female partner being there). A halo effect may have been present, with MSMW reporting an agreement type other than what was actually true in order to rationalize their sexual risk behaviors with other men outside of their relationship (i.e., reporting non-monogamous agreements with their partners, even though no such agreements were made). However, we purposely used an anonymous survey design to help decrease measurement error and participant bias [24].

In addition, individual-level data were collected only from the men in each relationship. Dyadic data would be much more informative. Such data would show how both partners understand their agreements and whether both partners operate under the same precise agreement. A final limitation might have been the demographic makeup of the sample itself. The men were predominately White, well educated, and relatively wealthy. Ironically, this sample actually may provide more novel data than if the sample had been more diverse racially. Previous research with MSMW has almost exclusively focused on sexual risk behaviors among minority populations, particularly African Americans [9, 19, 20, 25, 26]. Largely White populations have been studied far less.

Future social science research should be conducted to correct these limitations. Additionally, future research that focuses on dyadic data (e.g., information from both partners) is needed to measure the level of awareness that relational partners of MSMW have of their same-sex behaviors. Research that examines how relational and societal factors may inhibit or facilitate an individual's ability to discuss his or her sexual needs, including the preferred type of relationship and establishment of a sexual agreement, is urgently needed among MSMW relationships. Finally, the push for universal HIV testing in the United States and abroad may enhance awareness and provide a structural mechanism to instigate sexual health communication between couples.

Implications for social science

This research was merely one instance showing how a social science perspective can provide different insights into public health. Where more traditional epidemiologic studies focus on deficit-based models regarding at-risk populations (e.g., drug use leading to HIV risk in gay men), social science tests innovative social interaction- and relationship-based predictors that help to more precisely define and understand the intricacies of populations. As shown by the research, investigating aspects of the relationship can help illuminate the unique dynamics that may exist between partners and how public health programs can intervene to address these issues. For example, our main goal was to explore the sexual risk behaviors and relationship characteristics among MSMW; however, our study revealed inconsistent testing behaviors, inconsistent condom use, and the disconnect between what MSMW reported about their same-sex behaviors and what they reported about their agreements formed with their steady female partners.

Another positive aspect of using a social science research perspective (and shown by the present research) is the encouragement of more nuanced groupings within populations. Public health and epidemiological studies often focus on race/ethnicity, age, occupations, geographic areas, socioeconomic status, gender, and sexual orientation to indicate differences between individuals. In contrast, social science offers categorizations within populations that group men and women by their social identities, social networks, individual differences on social variables, and, as exemplified by the current study, subtypes of relationships. In short, a social frame placed on health research increases the external validity of studies' findings. Arguably, it is more likely that individuals would, in reality, self-categorize under such social categories rather than the more rigid, demographic ones suggested by epidemiology.

As a concluding point, social science research into health problems can help provide support for public health programs and interventions. Universal HIV/STI testing has been hotly debated over the past few years. The encouragement of primary care physicians to test everyone, regardless of obvious risk factors, remains controversial; however, social-based research studies, such as the present research, provide evidence for why such a change in protocol may be necessary. The sample of MSMW described in this study happens to be in dire need of a structural intervention, such as universal HIV/STI testing. As previously mentioned, it may be too stigmatizing or deleterious for the relationship for the men to communicate to their female partners either their extra-dyadic sexual encounters or their need to be HIV/STI tested. It is certain that future social science research studies will continue to provide evidence for the most efficacious interventions for at-risk groups, such as MSMW and their female partners.

Acknowledgments

This manuscript was supported by the center (P30-MH52776) and NRSA (T32-MH19985) grants from the National Institute of Mental Health. Special thanks are extended to the participants for their time and effort.

References

[1] CDC Prevalence and awareness of HIV infection among men who have sex with men, 21 Cities, United States, 2008. *MMWR* 2010; 59(37):1201-7.

[2] Coates TJ. What is to be done? *AIDS* 2008;22:1079–80.

[3] CDC. HIV in the United States, 2010. Accessed 2011 Oct 27. URL: http://www.cdc.gov/hiv/resources/factsheets/us.htm.

[4] CDC. HIV/AIDS and Women, 2007. Accessed 2011 Oct 27. URL: http://www.cdc.gov/hiv/topics/women/overview_partner.htm.

[5] Chu SY, Peterman TA, Doll LS, Buehler JW, Curran JW. AIDS in bisexual men in the United States: Epidemiology and transmission in women. *Am. J. Public Health 1992*;82:220-4.

[6] Kahn JG, Gurvey J, Pollack LM, Binson D, Catania JA. How many HIV infections cross the bisexual bridge? An estimate from the United States. *AIDS* 1997;11:1031-7.

[7] O'Leary A, Jones KT. Bisexual men and heterosexual women: How big is the bridge? How can we know? *Sex Transm. Dis.* 2006;33:594-5.

[8] Prabhu R, Owen CL, Folger K, McFarland W. The bisexual bridge revisited: Sexual risk behavior among men who have sex with men and women, San Francisco, 1998-2003. *AIDS* 2004;18:1604-6.

[9] Siegel K, Schrimshaw EW, Lekas H, Parsons JT. Sexual behaviors of non-gay identified non-disclosing men who have sex with men and women. *Arch. Sex Behav.* 2008;37:720-35.

[10] Wood RW, Krueger LE, Pearlman TC, Goldbaum G. HIV transmission: Women's risk from bisexual men. *Am. J. Public* Health 1993;83:1757-9.

[11] Zule WA, Bobashev GV, Wechsberg WM, Costenbader EC, Coomes CM. Behaviorally bisexual men and their risk behaviors with men and women. *J. Urban Health* 2009;86(1):S48-S62.

[12] Agronick G, O'Donnell L, Stueve A, Doval AS, Duran R, Vargo S. Sexual behaviors and risks among bisexually and gay-identified young Latino men. *AIDS Behav.* 2004;8:185-97.

[13] CDC. HIV/STD risks in young men who have sex with men who do not disclose their sexual orientation-Six U.S. cities, 1994-2000. *MMWR* 2003;52:81-5.

[14] Doll LS, Peterson LR, White CR, Johnson ES, Ward JW, The Blood Donor Study Group. Homosexuality and nonhomosexuality identified men who have sex with men: A behavioral comparison. *J. Sex Res.* 1992;29:1-14.

[15] Goldbaum G, Perdue T, Wolitski R, Rietmeijer C, Hedrich A, Wood R, et al. Differences in risk behavior and sources of AIDS information among gay, bisexual, and straight-identified men who have sex with men. *AIDS Care* 1998;12:13-21.

[16] Stokes JP, Vanable P, McKirnan DJ. Comparing gay and bisexual men on sexual behavior, condom use, and psychosocial variables related to HIV/AIDS. *Arch. Sex Behav.* 1997;26:383-97.

[17] Wold C, Seage GR, Lenderking WR, Mayer KH, Cai B, Heeren T, et al. Unsafe sex in men who have sex with both men and women. *J. Acquir Immune Defic Syndr* 1998;17:361-7.

[18] Jeffries WL. Sociodemographic, sexual, and HIV and other sexually transmitted disease risk profiles of nonhomosexual-identified men who have sex with men. *Am. J. Public Health* 2009;99:1042-5.

[19] Dodge B, Jeffries WL, Sandfort TGM. Beyond the down low: Sexual risk, protection, and disclosure among at-risk black men who have sex with both men and women (MSMW). *Arch. Sex Behav.* 2008;37:683-96.

[20] Washington TA, Wang Y, Browne D. Difference in condom use among sexually active males at historically black colleges and universities. *J Am Coll Health* 2009;57:411-8.

[21] Jeffries WL, Dodge B. Male bisexuality and condom use at last sexual encounter: Results from a national survey. *J. Sex Res.* 2007;44:278-89.

[22] Jeffries WL. HIV testing among bisexual men in the United States. *AIDS Educ. Prev.* 2010:22;356-370.

[23] Vittinghoff E, Douglas J, Judson F, McKirnan D, MacQueen K, Buchbinder SP. Per-contact risk of human immunodeficiency virus transmission between male sexual partners. *Am. J. Epidemiol.* 1999;150:306-11.

[24] Catania JA, Gibson DR, Chitwood DD, Coates TJ. Methodological problems in AIDS behavioral research: Influences on measurement error and participation bias in studies of sexual behavior. *Psychol. Bull* 1990;108:339-62.

[25] Millet G, Malebranche D, Mason B, Spikes P. Focusing "down low": bisexual black men, HIV risk and heterosexual transmission. *J. Natl. Med. Assoc.* 2005;97(Suppl 7):52S-9.

[26] Reback CJ, Larkins S. Maintaining a heterosexual identity: Sexual meanings among a sample of heterosexually identified men who have sex with men. *Arch. Sex Behav.* 2010;39:766-73.

In: Human Immunodeficiency Virus …
Editors: Hugh Klein and Joav Merrick
ISBN: 978-1-62081-293-8

Chapter V

Refashioning stigma: Experiencing and managing HIV/AIDS in the biomedical era

Yordanos Mequanint Tiruneh*
Department of Sociology, Northwestern University, Evanston, Illinois, US

Abstract

This chapter explores the stigma experiences of people living with HIV/AIDS (PLWHA) and evaluates the impact of antiretroviral treatment (ART) on their (a) lived experiences and (b) illness management. Qualitative research for this study is based on 105 in-depth interviews and ethnographic observation conducted between May and October of 2008 at an urban HIV clinic in a teaching hospital in Addis Ababa, Ethiopia. A phenomenological approach to data analysis isolated socio-cultural meanings underlying empirical variations of stigma experiences and examined how the availability of treatment alters the experience of living with chronic stigmatized diseases. The study reveals that ART can effect a physical and social rebirth with a renewed sense of self-worth that, together, improve the negative self-concept people develop following an HIV diagnosis. The study also demonstrates that stigma attached to HIV/AIDS remains pervasive in the era of ART. Indeed, ART creates new stigma concerns related to healthcare practices that arise when patients refill prescriptions and follow up on their treatment. This refashioned nature of stigma demands that we identify patterns of change in the perception, experience, and management of the illness. Identifying and analyzing sources of stigma for PLWHA allows us to isolate stigma triggers and devise structural changes that can reform elements of healthcare institutions that intensify HIV stigma. Such research is particularly important in resource-poor settings where the AIDS crisis lingers and the socio-cultural factors that influence the outcomes of intervention strategies require attention.

* Correspondence: Yordanos Mequanint Tiruneh, Department of Sociology, Northwestern University, 1810 Chicago Avenue, Evanston, IL 60208 United States. E-mail: yordanos@u. northwestern.edu or yordanosnu@gmail.com

Introduction

AIDS is one of the leading causes of morbidity and mortality among adults in Ethiopia. In 2005, the cumulative number of AIDS deaths was 1,267,000 with a projection to reach 1.9 million in 2010 [1]. AIDS accounted for 34% of young adult deaths, of which 66.3% occurred in urban areas [1]. It is estimated that, from 2000 to 2015, AIDS will increase mortality by 6% and reduce the population by 16% compared with what would have occurred in the absence of the disease [2]. Likewise, the average life expectancy in Ethiopia is 45.5 years, a figure that is estimated to decrease by 15% due to AIDS from 2010 to 2015 [2]. The anticipated universal coverage of ART, however, is assumed to reduce AIDS mortality by 41% compared to a projection without treatment and decrease the reduction in life expectancy due to HIV/AIDS [1]. Stigma is one of the major social drivers of the epidemic in Ethiopia, hindering early diagnosis and disclosure of one's HIV serostatus [3]. Stigma is rooted in the ignorance, cultural and religious beliefs, poverty, and fear that surround the disease [4]. This fear imposes a huge burden on efforts to contain the epidemic and care for PLWHA [4].

Since January 2005, Highly Active Antiretroviral Therapy (HAART) has been available to PLWHA in Ethiopia, free of charge, through the national ART program, which is supported by various national and international initiatives [5]. Across the country, 45,595 people had started treatment by the end of July, 2006, of which 47% were adult males and 48% were adult females [5]. The availability of ART in resource-poor settings generates a significant hope to reconstruct HIV as a chronic manageable condition and reduce the stigma that has been associated with HIV [6, 7]. ART's capacity to relieve or improve many symptoms of HIV infection, thereby restoring health and productivity and facilitating social integration [6], allows PLWHA to escape detection and the accompanying stigma that others associate with those who have the disease.

However, few studies have explored the lived experiences of those following biomedical management of the disease since HIV treatments have become available in such resource-poor settings [1, 2]. The relationship between stigma concerns of PLWHA and ART is among the lived experiences that require attention. HIV/AIDS is a disease that is often identified with "immoral" behavior and is perceived as contagious and threatening to the public. Furthermore, its contraction is often viewed as having been brought on by the diseased individual [8, 9]. For these reasons, HIV/AIDS is more highly stigmatized than other illnesses such as cancer [10], SARS, or tuberculosis [11]. Studying HIV stigma in a range of socio-cultural and political settings is imperative if we hope to understand the differential experiences of PLWHA [7, 12]. Ethiopia represents such a setting, as it exhibits all the abovementioned stigma concerns associated with socio-cultural and political environments. Indeed, because HIV is transmitted by socially produced behaviors that occur in specific social contexts, the experience and management of the disease is similarly context specific [13]. Therefore, although almost everyone living with HIV faces some form of stigma, the lived experiences and illness management practices of PLWHA in disparate socio-cultural contexts are affected differentially precisely because socio-cultural context affects the particular forms and triggers of stigma that occur.

In his classical work on stigma, which now forms the basis of most stigma studies, Erving Goffman defines stigma as a powerfully discrediting attribute that changes individuals' perception of the self and how they are viewed by others [14]. Although

Goffman did not have AIDS in mind when he defined stigma, scholars agree that HIV involves all three types of Goffman's stigmatized attributes: physical imperfection caused by progressive opportunistic infections, behavioral flaws characterized by moral transgression, and affliction through membership in a social group considered a "risk group" (e.g., commercial sex workers, IV drug users, and people with socially devalued sexual behaviors) [15]. Based on this classic definition, Alonzo et al. defined stigma as the construction of a deviation from the "normal" due to undesirable or distinguishing attributes that impose a risk of isolation from the self as well as society [8]. HIV stigma is a social construct that is rooted in the far larger conceptualizations of gender, sexuality, race, class, and culture. Its salience rises and falls throughout the illness trajectory because the attributes that trigger stigma can be concealed at some stages of the illness but not in others. Moreover, the targets of stigma vary across cultures, and are uniquely experienced by each person depending on the social environment and the nature of the stigmatizing condition [8, 10]. Holzemer et al. point to the cyclic nature of HIV stigma. Stigma begins with a trigger (HIV testing, illness symptoms, or filling a prescription) that leads to negative health outcomes (such as suboptimal treatment adherence and disease progression), that, in turn, become triggers in their own right [16].

Extant research concerning stigma in the context of HIV yields several observations: First, HIV is an extraordinarily unique illness with universal, multi-dimensional stigmatization that can arise immediately following a diagnosis, at the appearance of symptoms, and even because it is still considered untreatable by many people [8, 10]. Second, PLWHA often experience social rejection, isolation, economic discrimination, blame, and a negative self-concept [10, 17]. Third, HIV stigma is persistent in spite of our better understanding of the disease and the advent of successful treatment options [18], and efforts to reduce stigma have been met with only moderate success [19]. Few studies afford provisional support to the link between stigma reduction and ART provision [20, 21] while others challenge the argument that availability of treatment reduces stigma [22, 23]. Fourth, stigma negatively affects the success of effective HIV prevention and care efforts (including adherence to prescribed medical regimens). Most studies indicate that the greater the stigma the more consistently it is associated with missed doses of prescribed medications, medication non-adherence, and poor health outcomes [24–28].

A review of the relevant literature exposes two gaps. First, not many studies have examined stigma from the sufferers' perspectives using their lived experiences to anchor the analysis [7, 15]. Second, only a few studies have been conducted to examine how HIV treatment has reshaped the public conceptualization of HIV/AIDS and how stigma affects illness management on the part of PLWHA [20-23]. By examining the lived experiences and illness management of PLWHA, this qualitative study examines the dynamic relationship between HIV treatment and stigma, three years after free provision of ART in an urban setting in Ethiopia. It is both important and timely to examine how ART has refashioned HIV stigma, particularly in resource-poor settings like Ethiopia where the AIDS crisis is still rampant and the impacts of ART remain recent and, largely, unknown.

The study

This chapter is part of a larger project that explores the lived experiences and illness management of PLWHA in Ethiopia. The overall goal of the study was to understand how PLWHA in Ethiopia perceive, experience, and manage their illness in the era of effective HIV treatment. The study was conducted in an urban HIV/AIDS clinic at a teaching hospital in Addis Ababa, Ethiopia. Consistent with trends seen in most metropolitan areas in developing countries, Addis is characterized by extreme socio-economic and cultural contrasts, with a few modern sectors that are relatively technologically advanced by Western standards and many others that remain culturally traditional. The city is further characterized by extreme socioeconomic polarization, with huge income disparities between a few millionaires and most others, who struggle for daily survival. It is the most diverse city in Ethiopia, attracting people representing a range of cultures and ethnicities from all over the country, including a recently urbanized rural population that has migrated to the big city in search of jobs. This rural-urban exodus coupled with the continuously growing population in such a limited economy escalates unemployment, overburdens the city's poorly developed infrastructure, and engenders widespread ghettos that exhibit all the vices associated with urban poverty.

This urban setting was chosen as the research site for several epidemiological and social reasons. First, HIV is highly prevalent in and inflicts considerable social and economic impacts on urban areas. For instance, two-thirds (66.3%) of all urban deaths of people between the ages of 15 and 49 are due to AIDS [4]. Second, Addis exhibits a relatively high rate of people living with HIV (11.5%), and houses several HIV treatment sites [4]. Third, as already noted, Addis is characterized by a great diversity of ethnicities, socioeconomic statuses, religions, and worldviews. And, fourth, in Addis traditionalism and modernism simultaneously inform all aspects of life. All of these societal factors shape the contexts in which PLWHA construct their social identities and their choices of illness-management strategies. This complex admixture of societal factors facilitated the selection of a diverse participant sample, revealing the realities of life for PLWHA as anything but monolithic.

Since the literature contains no sociological studies of the illness experiences of people living with HIV in the study area, the present research employs a qualitative approach suited to the examination of phenomena that otherwise are inaccessible through comprehensive scientific investigation. Between May and October of 2008, six months of ethnographic observation and interviews were conducted at St. Michael's hospital, which facilitated obtaining a rich, exploratory account of individual experiences and actual practices that would be unattainable through quantitative investigation. In-depth interviews were conducted with 105 PLWHA who were selected randomly during their clinic visits. To form the sample, clinic nurses chose every other or every third patient (depending on the total number of patients on a given day) to inform potential participants about the research. The researcher then approached those who agreed to participate in the study to explain its purpose and procedures in detail. The researcher obtained informed consent from the participants after a thorough explanation and clarification of the study's nature, purpose, and potential risk.

To take part in the study, participants had to satisfy the following criteria: being 18 years of age or older, having begun antiretroviral therapy at least six months prior to the study, and experiencing no acute/serious symptoms of illness at the time of the interview. Acute illness was added as a criterion of exclusion because interviewing sick people potentially raised two ethical issues: First, information given by sick participants might be unreliable and incomplete, simply because of the strain of being interviewed, threatening the study's scientific rigor. Second, approaching potential research subjects who were acutely ill would be inconsiderate and might increase their suffering. Such exclusion of potential participants might introduce bias in the data insofar as acutely sick people might view their illness and illness management differently from those whose symptoms are milder or no longer present. However, over the course of the interviews, several accounts of participants' experiences with acute symptoms of the illness were elicited by probing relatively healthier subjects to reflect on times when they had been very sick. Consequently, applying acute illness as an exclusion criterion did not significantly compromise the study.

All of the interviews were conducted in one of the examination rooms in the clinic, which provided a private space for a confidential exchange. Each interview was completed with collection of socio-demographic information. To protect confidentiality, case numbers were assigned to each participant. Ethical approvals were obtained from the Northwestern University Institutional Review Board, Addis Ababa University, Medical Faculty, Institutional Review Board, and the Ethiopian Science and Technology Agency.

The interviews averaged 75 minutes in length, with none running beyond two hours, and were conducted in Amharic by the researcher, a native speaker. The interview guide supported the gathering of information on typical days in their lives; their relationships with families, friends, and neighbors; what it means to them to spend time with people in their social networks; their social lives before and after an HIV-positive diagnosis; and how they navigate their relationships with and responsibilities for others while undergoing HIV treatment. After providing unprompted descriptions of their experiences of stigma in response to the aforementioned questions, participants were asked a direct question about whether or not they had experienced stigma due to their HIV serostatus. The majority of the stigma data were obtained through the former, unprompted questions, rather than from the one specifically about stigma. The direct question on stigma yielded minimal data, usually related to external experiences of stigma, mostly enacted. Then the stigma experiences of PLWHA were examined using an interpretive phenomenological approach in order to understand how the social world inhabited by individuals living with HIV contributes to similarities and differences in their stigma experiences. With this approach, it was possible to elicit more than subjective descriptions of experiences, revealing meanings embedded in the lived experiences of PLWHA that in some cases are not apparent to the participants themselves [29]. Moreover, phenomenology makes it possible to explore stigma experiences from the individual perspectives of PLWHAs based on their lived experiences.

All of the interviews were recorded and translated into English, and then analyzed using phenomenological methods to explore the meanings of peoples' experiences [29]. Investigating interviewees' phenomenology entailed probing their perceptions of their experiences as ART recipients to elicit from them the meanings they attach to their subjective experiences of "living with HIV." This entailed asking them to express their feelings about and reactions to taking their medications as well as following their medical regimens and the associated recommendations (such as dose schedules and dietary prescriptions). Participants were also asked to share their perceptions of the outcomes of treatment and of their overall experience with managing their medications in their respective social worlds in their daily lives. This method is intended to capture the meanings of participants' lived experiences based on reflective description of those experiences on the part of the people themselves within their familiar social contexts. In this way the researcher was able to explore the participants' worlds as perceived in their narratives and understand how these perceived meanings shape and organize peoples' experiences as they live with HIV/AIDS. Interview transcripts and field notes were coded carefully using HyperResearch qualitative software. Perspectives identified by similar codes were compared and categorized into groups. Emergent themes were identified and related to people's socio-cultural perception and experiences of living with HIV in the era of biomedical treatment and its impact on illness management. The results of these analyses are reported below.

Findings

The study site served a diverse population at the time the research was conducted (see Table 1). Among the total of 105 study participants, 62 (59%) were women. The mean age of the participants was 37.7 years; their ages ranged from 21 to 58 years. The length of time since participants had started ART ranged from 6 to 76 months (mean=31.6 months). Thirty-nine (37.1%) were single, whereas 31 (29.5%) were married, 18 (17.1%) were widowed, and 17 (16.2%) were separated/divorced. Only 15 (14.3%) of the participants had studied at the college level, whereas 47 (44.7%) had elementary education or had also attended but did not graduate from high school. Thirteen (12.4%) of the participants were illiterate (could not read or write). Sixty-six (62.9%) were Orthodox Christians. There were 18 Protestants (17.1%) and 13 Muslims (12.4 %). More than two-thirds of the participants (74, comprising 70.4%) had no income or led a very impoverished life with marginal incomes of less than 500 birr per month (equivalent to $50).

More than ninety percent (91.4%) of the 105 participants mentioned having experienced stigma. These experiences varied widely in both type and degree. The degree of stigma experienced was greater among people who admitted that they contracted the disease due to their own risk-taking behavior than it was among those who felt they had no control over the acquisition of the disease (e.g., it was contracted following a medical procedure or while being confined in prison or a refugee camp). In either case, the stigma attached to HIV/AIDS is still pervasive in the era of effective treatment. Since the HIV epidemic in Ethiopia is not associated with homosexuality or IV drug use, social identity did not stand out in explaining differential stigma experiences at the macro level. At the micro level, however, HIV is associated closely with morality and evil [8], and most of the stigma concerns are rooted in the dominant moral discourses surrounding HIV.

In particular, these discourses characterize HIV as being a product of deviations from sexual moralities [30] and, in the context of this study set in Ethiopia, this means having multiple sexual partners or being adulterous. The lived experiences of PLWHA taking ART in Ethiopia was characterized by a complex ongoing struggle of, on the one hand, managing stigma and, on the other, following HIV treatment as prescribed. This study illustrates how ART lessens certain types of stigma while augmenting others and creates new stigma triggers that PLWHA had never had to negotiate before the medication's roll-out. By identifying these associations between ART and stigma, both positive and negative, the remainder of this section provides more detailed evidence of the lived experiences of PLWHA in the biomedical era.

Table 1. Sociodemographic characteristics of PLWHA (n=105)

Characteristics	Number
Sex	
Female	62
Age	
18–29	21
30–39	41
40–49	12
50 and above	31
Marital Status	
Married	31
Never Married	39
Divorced	7
Separated	10
Widowed	18
Have Children	
Yes	64
Educational Status	
Illiterate	13
Elementary	31
High School	16
High school/voc. school graduate	30
College education	15
Employment Status	
Employed in the formal sector	30
Self-employed	43
Unemployed	32
Monthly Income	
No income	18
No regular income	23
Under 500 birr (under $50)	33
500–1499 birr ($50–$150)	19
1500 birr and above (above $150)	12
Religion	
Orthodox Christian	66
Muslim	13
Protestant	18
Jehovah's Witness	3
ND Christian	3
No religion	2
Months on ART	
6–24	40
25–48	58
49 and above	7

Concealing Difference

ART is beneficial in concealing discreditable attributes associated with HIV/AIDS by improving biomedical conditions and combating stereotypical bodily symptoms associated with the disease. Many PLWHA using ART mentioned feeling healthy, being able to resume functional daily living, and needing less frequent clinic visits as countervailing factors that reduce the sense of "differentness" and negative self-concept that typically accompany an HIV-positive diagnosis. The following quotes emphasize several respects in which normalcy is restored following improved health conditions:

> Everybody expected me to die. After I started the medicine and as I got well physically, I guess people started to even doubt whether we [my wife and I] have the virus or not for certain. (Male, 47)

> Now, there is nothing that I worry about. I am happy, as people who didn't shake hands with me before embrace me today. People have started to give me the right treatment . . . . Before I started the treatment, I had stopped going to social gatherings, but now I go to weddings, funerals, and I am active in social life. (Female, 58)

> I am working, doing what everybody else is doing. If I were inferior to other healthy people, say if I were bedridden, I would have been scared. But now I am not worried. I am healthy now, and I got all my confidence back. (Female, 29)

As these quotes suggest, a second way in which medical treatments restore normalcy is through bringing back functional competence and helping people regain social and economic liberation, vital quality-of-life interests that once were threatened by the illness. Opportunistic illnesses that prevented PLWHA from working were major stigma triggers that were often intensified by corresponding stigma associated with being economically dependent. Perceived HIV stigma was reduced for PLWHA by improved functional status (expressed in terms of functional activity and the ability to participate in the labor force), as many interviewees had been bedridden or seriously ill before treatment. Consequently, some PLWHA reported having built a strong positive relationship with their medication (calling it a friend, a lover, a supporter, or a partner), which enables them to fight against impending physical as well as social death (stigma) and promises better health and social rebirth.

Creating support

Pill taking also resulted in the creation of substitute social networks with promising social capital that were helpful in supporting illness management and coping with stigma. Such networks were created naturally when PLWHA met at HIV clinics for follow-up appointments or to refill their prescriptions, or artificially through support groups created by civic organizations (non-governmental organizations and patient organizations). Such relationships persisted beyond the settings in which they were formed and naturally created networks often last longer than do those created in artificially organized support groups. These new relationships facilitated the exchange of material resources (money, food, shelter) as well as non-material resources (information, encouragement) and acceptance of health status among people undergoing medical treatment. Additionally, they helped PLWHA develop a sense of belongingness, and construct a collective identity borne of HIV-tainted blood. This sense of collective identity is illustrated by one participant as follows:

> The medication has earned me a lot of friends. People who come from different Kifle Ketemas [the lowest administrative unit in Ethiopia, equivalent to a county] meet here. A person who takes ART and a prisoner is the same. We take care of each other . . . like prisoners take care of each other. The same is true with people who take the medication . . . . We help each other. (Male, 40)

Such anecdotes highlight the unintended positive consequences of ART that tended to ameliorate the affects of disease stigmatization. That they were facilitated by institutions and circumstances that would not exist in the absence of ART suggests how beneficial outcomes might materialize from otherwise bad situations.

Medication as stigma trigger

Although ART is perceived as enabling PLWHA to conceal differences and create social ties, the regimen management it entails often generates external stigma by publicizing what Goffman [14] characterized as discreditable attributes (HIV status per se, and the physical changes associated with treatment, bring discredit to the sufferer). In some cases undergoing ART actually reinforces stigma by reminding PLWHA that they are possessors of these discredited attributes. HIV treatment imposes stigma concerns at various levels of regimen management. The most frequently mentioned stigma trigger is the location and configuration of health care facilities, as PLWHA often wished not to be associated with the clinics from which they obtained services. Most of the participants in this study, for example, were not comfortable with the location of the HIV clinic they had to use. Their HIV clinic was segregated from other infectious disease clinics and made it difficult for patients to maintain their privacy. Service notices that were commonly posted on doors, walls, and notice boards indicated the clinic's purpose. By Western standards of privacy for PLWHA, the HIV clinics in Ethiopia are far less equipped to maintain the privacy of individuals. The following quotes demonstrate how the PLWHA in this study feared exposure due to the physical structure of ART clinics:

> This has been repeatedly said; the location of the HIV clinic is very embarrassing. One time, I met a friend around the waiting area, and while I was talking with him, it was my turn and my name was called. He then knew about my status. (Male, 37)

> I mean, you see everybody who is attending this clinic; it is kind of out in the open and people obviously know what this clinic is for. I do not believe the clinic is doing a great job in serving us confidentially given the location. (Female, 29)

Long wait times at the clinic and certain procedures that PLWHA needed to follow to refill their prescriptions were reported as stigma triggers, potentially threatening regimen recommendations. After all, PLWHA in Ethiopia know that being HIV-positive is a sufficient source of stigma once one's HIV status is known, so being exposed as such in public triggers that stigma. Another participant described his clinic experience in these terms:

> Sometimes, it is difficult to come here, line up with other people, and take the medication. Recently, it is getting better. [Before], there was a need to line up for three or four hours to take the medication. People do not want to be seen by other people who come to get treatments for other sicknesses; people might be afraid. These things push many people living with the virus to stop taking the medication. (Male, 38)

Some even argued that the "differentness" and deviancy identified with HIV was reinforced by the medical profession itself, because, generally, HIV clinics were segregated from other infectious disease clinics and involve special paperwork and procedures of operation: "I would have been very happy if HIV is treated like other illnesses. I do not see the reason to have a separate clinic for HIV if we are seen like any other patient" (Female, 29). Many participants mentioned their concerns about stigma resulting from following routine clinical procedures, such as taking their charts to the pharmacy. A patient explained:

> The [HIV-positive patient's] chart has a unique cover that makes it different from other patients' charts. That difference by itself makes you liable to peoples' gossip. I often see people hiding their charts under their shirts or putting them in a plastic bag when they take them to the pharmacy. I sometimes offer to take other peoples' charts along with mine when I see their discomfort. (Female, 25)

Outside of the clinic setting, stigma concerns extended to the handling of pills—transporting medication, storing medication at home, and discarding empty pill bottles. Public familiarity with ART heightened the disclosure concerns of PLWHA. As one patient explained,

> People recognize the medication. It is better these days. Earlier it[pill bottle] even had a logo on it, you know, the red ribbon, the HIV logo. It [ART] can be identified. Now the bottle doesn't have such a mark, but people have already associated that particular bottle with HIV medicine, even if it is not . . . (Male, 29)

In some cases, internalized fear of disclosure escalated to a remarkable degree of obsession and paranoia. The following excerpt demonstrates the magnitude of such fear and the conflicting pressures that some PLWHA experienced in an effort to normalize and conceal their situation:

> The great majority of the public is informed about ART. People know and could identify the ART tablet. If you are once noticed taking ART, you will be automatically labeled as "HIV" . . . I am not even comfortable leaving my pills at home. I put on a big jacket and I keep all my pills in my pocket . . . . No one can tell what is inside my pocket. For this reason I refill my prescription strictly on a monthly basis. This is because I do not feel safe to leave my pills at home . . . . If something unexpected happens, for instance, if a fire breaks out in a nearby house and extends to other houses in the neighborhood, people might end up seeing my pills in an effort to control the fire. Also, the door of my house is made of a corrugated iron sheet. The space in between the joints of the door provides easy access to look into what is in the room. (Male, 47)

This example demonstrates the diversity of lived experiences of PLWHA in contrasting socio-cultural settings. Here, the patient is explicitly concerned with the stigma he will suffer, whereas in a wealthy country the discovery of pills is most commonly associated with the fear that others might find them, take them, and harm themselves.

People with HIV who traveled frequently and were obliged to take their doses outside their homes also cited packaging and the number of pills to be taken per dose/day as a stigma concern:

> If only one tablet was taken, it would be easy to just carry one in a small container or something, but taking three different tablets makes it difficult to be discreet. It is packed in a big bottle, and it is noisy, too. Some people drop the whole container when they try to hide it. And for people who travel a lot it is even more difficult. (Male, 40)

Another woman also mentioned her stigma concern related to packaging:

> My pills have a huge potential to stigmatize me. That is why, for instance, every time I refill my prescription, I transfer all the pills in another container as I don't want people to see the original package, which is also cumbersome and noisy. (Female, 50)

The second way in which pill taking augmented an internalized negative self-concept lies in the visible physical changes that were observed after a severe illness, which, in the case of PLWHA, was felt as an indirect confirmation of their HIV status. Such physical changes can either be positive (improving an individual's appearance) or negative (creating visible symptoms of medication side effects that further served as stigma triggers by highlighting physical imperfections). The following quote illustrates how negative physical changes after treatment became a visual cue to stigma:

> I lost everything. I became slim and looked like a man. No curves at all. I went to my doctor and cried because I was so upset that I was not told about the side effects. The doctor said that the side effect was only alteration of a body shape, which is not life threatening and she did not think it is important to inform me. Imagine how it could be psychologically traumatic for a single young woman like me to live with this new physique. It is better to die. What is bad about dying? It is much better than living with this body shape. It is really disgusting to have your body shape disproportioned all of a sudden. To make the situation worse, everybody that I know asks me what happened to me as the change was so noticeable. (Female, 29)

The final way in which pill taking augmented negative self-concept was by reminding PLWHA of their status as HIV-positive, and devaluing them as inferior and dependent on medication for normal functioning. The following quote illustrates how some people internalize a negative self-concept from being dependent on pills:

> When I think of the two tablets that keep me alive, I hate myself and I feel that I am dead. Sometimes I get furious to see myself like a walking corpse, and other times I see myself as a doll that functions with a battery. I would say, without these batteries [pills], I am nothing. (Male, 50)

In some cases, pills triggered a sense of internalized blame for contracting the disease. For people who assumed total personal responsibility for contracting the virus, pill taking was the price that they had to pay for their unfortunate mistakes. "When I take my medication, I always think of the moment I made a mistake [had casual sex]," one participant explained (Female, 30). Pill taking may also play a symbolic role in lowered expectations, perceptions of vulnerability, and dependence on others, even among people who know of their HIV serostatus.

Management of medication-induced stigma

The interview data revealed that PLWHA were engaged on a constant basis in concealment work to assert normalcy and conceal discreditable attributes or indicators that serve as stigma triggers, such as pill taking. The following quote shows the engagement with both impression and information management that is typical of PLWHA:

> The reason why many people, especially those who live in a house rented from private owners, stop their medication is that they are afraid of being identified with the medicine [1]. Even when they go to the hospital regularly, people are careful not to set a noticeable pattern and be suspected that their visit was to refill their ART. Most people hate to take their medication from a nearby hospital or health center, as people living in the same locality go to the same health institutions and chances of being identified is high. For example, PLWHA living in my surroundings don't want to get their HIV treatment from St. John [hospital pseudonym] for the hospital serves people from our neighborhood. A person who runs into someone from his neighborhood won't show up to the hospital again and will discontinue taking the medication . . . . For all these reasons, many discontinue their medication. (Female, 41)

Concealment work included silence, hiding/passing as "normal," lying, skipping a dose, and even stopping medication entirely. Most PLWHA emphasized that they literally lied about or hid their medication from most people in their social network. As one man explained,

> I am keeping it secret because of the stigma. Otherwise, if it were diabetes, I would have said I have diabetes. If it was diabetes pills, I would definitely have taken it differently. I am talking to you now because you are a professional. Otherwise, I do not want anybody to know that I am HIV-positive. If people ask me about my pills, I would say I am diabetic or hypertensive. I will never say that I have HIV. The stigma is still strong. (Male, 49)

---

[1] The social context of renting a house from a private landlord in Ethiopia differs from that of the West on physical, cultural, and legal grounds. When private landlords rent their houses, it is done mostly as a unit (an addition or a separate room) that they are subletting. In most cases the landlord lives in the same compound, which automatically increases the intensity and frequency of interaction with the tenants. Such congested housing arrangements, especially in inner cities, inevitably compromise privacy. In addition to the physical proximity of the dwelling units, the communal life in Ethiopia that fairly demands socialization with neighbors, including landlords, allows the latter to intrude into the private lives of their tenants. In most cases, there is no lease/contract to rent a house from a private landlord. The landlords can raise the rent, set limitations on the use of resources, and even evict a tenant whenever they want to, and there is no legal protection for tenants in place. Lack of such legal protections results in a hierarchical relationship between the landlord and the tenant, putting the latter in a disadvantaged position. The extreme fear of disclosure and stigma among people who rent houses from private landlords could be a reflection of the power gradient between PLWHA and their landlords.

PLWHA also strived constantly to conceal their status and diverted suspicion by passing as "normal" or doing things that they used to do before becoming ill, such as consuming alcohol or using drugs. Often, medication management was compromised when PLWHA were at work, engaged in leisure time, or were amid others in a social setting. In such instances, they avoided exposure, simply lied about diagnosis and treatment, or diverted attention from themselves while taking the medication. A woman described her effort to conceal her HIV status as follows:

> It is hard to keep this thing [HIV] under wraps, especially if you are seen at the clinic [HIV]. Thank goodness I haven't encountered anyone in a place where they can be sure of my diagnosis. If anyone sees me at any time, I will say that I came for a diabetes check up. People only know that I am diabetic. I once ran into my cousin, and when she asked me why I came here, I told her that I had my diabetic follow-up here [at the hospital]. I am always cautious. For fear of being noticed, I cover myself with my wraps all year long, wear sunglasses even if it is raining [laughter] . . . . It is hard. (Female, 50)

In the case of HIV, concealment work was frequently complicated by complex medication regimens. PLWHA's routines were dictated by their dose schedules. A woman described the demanding nature of managing stigma triggers as follows:

> When I have social commitments, or if I go to places where there is nothing to drink, I take my medication just with my saliva to be sure I take it on time. Now I am getting used to taking the drug without water. But whenever I plan to go somewhere, I always think about the people that I will be seeing; sometimes I will go after 10 o'clock, which is after taking my morning pills. The medication has taken spontaneity out of my life. This is such a depressing life. Sometimes I say to myself, for how long can I keep up with this hide-and-seek? But then again I fear . . . (Female, 30)

Frequently, self-exclusion, as a strategy to manage stigma, was intensified in an effort to manage internalized fears of disclosure. PLWHA avoided stigma triggers by voluntarily excluding themselves from available services or otherwise denying themselves opportunities for less-stigmatizing treatment alternatives. To minimize stigma triggers, PLWHA sometimes bought medication directly from a pharmacy, on the black market, or from poor patients who were desperate for money even if it meant risking their lives. Such behaviors persisted even while free treatment was offered at designated HIV clinics. The following quote illustrates this:

> A very rich man in my neighborhood came to my house, as everybody knows my status, and asked me to sell him my medication because he did not want to go to the clinic and get his treatment. This is because of fear of disclosure. Then I told him, "Listen, my CD4 count and yours may not be the same. Why don't you go to the clinic and get proper service? Also, I do not want to sell my medication and die. My life is as worthy as yours." He said, "You get three months worth of supply, so please sell two months of supply to me." I said no way. I told him that the medication is free, and he can go get it from the clinic. He mentioned his worries about being seen at the HIV clinic, and I reassured him that unless he discloses, no one would know about him just because he went to the clinic. He refused and said he would rather try the Holy water, and went to his hometown, only to die after a short while. (Female, 49)

This case indicates that, although experiencing "layered stigma" (stigma related to both poverty and HIV/AIDS) usually adds difficulty to the lives of PLWHA, HIV stigma also affects affluent people who are perhaps even more desperate to protect their privacy.

Self-exclusion based on access to medication affected the willingness not only to seek health services but also economic opportunities. Some PLWHA refrained from taking job offers that might make it difficult to avoid signaling their HIV status. As one participant explained,

> I love to work, and I don't even mind working as a daily laborer. But I don't want anyone to see my medication. For instance, I had an opportunity to be employed in a hair salon as stylist, but the owner told me that I would have to start work at 6:00 in the morning. That would have meant I couldn't take my medication at 8:00 because she would be around. So I declined the job offer. (Female, 31)

Social withdrawal was another common stigma management strategy that was employed within networks comprised of people who did not know their HIV serostatus. The rationale for social withdrawal was based on both disclosure concerns and health concerns. Existing networks may engage in certain normative activities (such as drinking alcohol) that may not be compatible with living with the virus. Yet withdrawal potentially intensified an internalized negative self-concept for the possessor, as she or he continued to be aware of being different [8]. As one participant explained,

> It is just confusing even for me. You know how it is. My inner self tells me to stay away. I don't know why but my personality has changed. I am easily irritable now. I became a complainer. I easily get upset. I was not like that, but now I have a short temper. When people chat with me, I get bored; I don't have much interest. (Male, 39)

Regardless of the various stigma management strategies used, there were times when stigma triggers were unavoidable. In such instances, PLWHA followed one of two schemata.

First, they might compromise their prescribed medication practices by skipping a dose or discontinuing treatment. Second, they might abandon information and impression management efforts and, instead, actively resist stigma through public HIV education and activism. Some adopted a more passive approach, simply learning to be less concerned about stigma. People who were economically independent, had supportive networks in which others accepted them and made them feel normal, or had experienced deteriorated health while attempting to manage stigma, were most likely to adopt passive stigma resistance.

Alternatively, people who lacked supportive networks, had no reliable means of subsistence, or experienced discrimination from people in their close network often engaged in active stigma resistance such as public advocacy or willful self-acceptance.

Together, then, these findings reveal how the advent of ART has changed the landscape of HIV stigmatization and how people variably managed stigma experiences in an era of effective treatment.

Discussion

Based on its findings that ART both helps and hinders stigma experiences and management of PLWHA, this study proposes an alternate directional pathway between stigma and disease/illness management. Unlike most previous studies that have focused on a single element of disease experience, the present study uniquely presents the lived experiences of PLWHA as they relate to both stigma and normalization. Integrating these two aspects of HIV experiences helps broaden the understanding of the complex experiences of people coping with HIV/AIDS, which, according to empirical studies [10, 11] as well as general theoretical formulations of stigma [13], qualifies as the most stigmatized disease across many cultures. The findings depict the various ways in which individuals suffer from stigma, including those that are attached to taking ART. The study also evinces ways in which ART enables individuals to achieve normalcy despite dealing with a chronic illness.

More specifically, the present study's findings indicate that ART restores a sense of normalcy in three ways. Primarily, as other research has found [8, 15, 23], ART improves a patient's biophysical trajectory directly or indirectly, which decreases stigma because physical imperfections (especially those stereotypically associated with the "HIV body") are minimized dramatically. Second, functional health status plays an important role in determining the degree to which people feel rejected socially [10]. In this way, ART targets the "layered stigma" [17] that PLWHA experience, not simply because of the immorality to which the acquisition of the disease is often attributed, but also because of its implicit association with other forms of negative social representations (such as nonproductive/dysfunctional status). In the face of massive poverty, PLWHA in Ethiopia have to navigate a socio-economic and political environment in which such factors, based largely on dependence, determines a community's response to HIV/AIDS. Indeed, rather than assuming that stigma leads patients to default on their medical treatment, this study demonstrates the opposite outcome in many cases, in which stigma leads to increased dedication to treatment, highlighting the necessity of examining stigma experiences within the broader social context.

A third way in which normalization through ART was observed in this study is coincidental to the treatment but also due to the role of clinics. PLWHA who must visit clinics in the course of treatment form networks outside of their existing social networks with other PLWHA. Relationships forged in this way, through a shared sense of differentness and vulnerability, soften and diffuse negative impacts of stigma experiences. Moreover, the organic nature of support groups formed naturally through clinical encounters may be even more instrumental in equipping patients with "tricks of the trade" [8] for concealing HIV status, coping with stigma, navigating resources, and (in some cases) coming out and resisting HIV-related stigma.

However, outside of ART's normalizing influence, other findings of this study are consistent with those of other studies in both developing and developed countries, suggesting that stigma partly explains poor adherence to ART [24–28, 31–34]. This study also supports stigma models in Africa [16] that demonstrate that HIV-related stigma among people undergoing ART sustain a vicious circle of illness for PLWHA. For a considerable number of participants in this study, internalized fear of disclosure was the main reason for treatment default and dose irregularity. This often led to worsening health conditions and, thereby, stimulated additional stigma concerns. This underscores the dilemma faced by PLWHA, whose health status is caught between the need to follow a treatment regimen as prescribed and the desire to conceal an HIV-positive status and pass as "normal." While it has been established that information-based awareness does not result in widespread reduction of stigma [35], the present study takes the argument one step further, asserting that factual information about stigmatized health conditions might lead to public identification of sufferers and subsequent stigmatization. Today, public awareness of the pills that are administered in ART has become a liability to individuals undergoing treatment.

This study has also provided evidence regarding attitudes toward pills in Ethiopian society, demonstrating that the salient association between pill taking and illness in Ethiopia results in particularly low expectations for positive outcomes that might result from taking pills. This finding confirms the argument in Alonzo et al [8] that lowered expectations formed out of sympathy (mostly within intimate networks) and extraordinary support are sometimes taken as expressions of stigma and vulnerability. In particular, in the context of the study area, pill taking is associated with being sick, unlike in the West, where pill taking is a relatively normal practice as people regularly consume vitamins, nutritional supplements, and common over-the-counter pain medications such as aspirin and ibuprofen. In Ethiopia, people who take pills regularly are presumed vulnerable to some debilitating condition, and often stigmatized for it. That is, most people in the study area believe that if you are taking pills something must be wrong with you.

The introduction of ART in resource-poor settings both increases and reduces HIV stigma at various junctures of the treatment process. This study echoes the views of other studies in poor settings that find that ART lessens stigma experiences that emanate from physical imperfections and socio-economic dependence [21, 23]; yet, it also increases the psychosocial vulnerability that PLWHA encounter at health facilities that augment other stigma experiences, and even create new stigma triggers that stem from the process of following medical regimens. In this regard, health institutions in African settings provide unique social spaces for contrasting cultural systems that consistently interact to frame and shape the behavior and illness management strategies of PLWHA. On the one hand, health facilities face the normalization of HIV as a manageable chronic condition as per conventional medicine and, on the other hand, they must acknowledge the complex social realities of AIDS and the distinctive pressures of HIV stigma in the African context. The differing nature of such findings indicates that in order to understand the dynamic and evolving illness management experiences of PLWHA, it is imperative to account for aspects of stigma and normalization as well as how people navigate and reconcile the two schemata.

In areas of high HIV prevalence, where stigma is still rampant and unintended disclosure is a serious issue, adherence to a prescribed regimen is a considerable challenge in spite of the treatment's capacity to restore self-worth. To overcome this challenge, HIV clinics should adopt policies and reconfigure facilities to provide due consideration for privacy. Measures to address challenges involved in accessing treatment and thereby reduce treatment default or lapses might include fewer personal identification procedures, waiting areas that reduce public exposure, decreased wait times, considerate and understanding health professionals who are attentive to the social context of PLWHA, and well-integrated care including mental health services. Similarly, concerns with frequency of dosage, pill size, and pill packaging undermine effective incorporation of medication into the daily lives of PLWHA.

Accordingly, dosage simplification and easy-to-handle packaging would facilitate the practicalities of following up on treatment in the face of a serious social risk of stigma.

In spite of these challenges, there are reasons for optimism independent of the opportunity to improve clinical facilities and engagement. The interview data collected in this study show that ideological resistance to the notion of "differentness" is expanding in the wake of ART's roll-out. PLWHA often abandon efforts related to information and impression management and start resisting stigma when they grow tired of the "hide and seek" drama of concealing their HIV status. Indeed, many who pervasively experience stigma are nevertheless encouraged by the outcomes of the medication and truly question the "discredit" attached to the disease when they consider that they are able to do whatever others are doing. Some such people depart from the vicious circle of stigma and decide to fight back against stigma triggers through actively teaching the public about HIV or, passively, by willfully reducing their stigma concerns. This finding reveals a wide variation in stigma experiences, which can be affected by PLWHA's general economic, identity, or social status. Considering how recently the scale-up of ART in Ethiopia began, the positive outcomes realized through the treatment might triumph over the stigma attached to HIV in the long run. However, much remains to be learned about the complex interplay between disease stigmatization and effective treatment in the context of poverty.

Overall, the findings of this study underscore the need to study such experiences at the individual level. Nonetheless, it also suggests the importance of extrapolating from individual experiences in order to seek more context-specific, comprehensive solutions (e.g., reconfiguring the structure of particular medical clinics or catering outreach to religious or prevailing cultural beliefs in localized areas). Many of these solutions might be structural in nature, demonstrating the benefits of such evidence-based studies that identify the social and structural drivers of poor health management by addressing underlying social conditions that interfere with proper prevention and treatment intervention approaches. Additionally, public health initiatives aimed at educating people about HIV/AIDS might address the stigma associated with the disease by encouraging patients to combat their negative and exhausting attempts at concealment by emphasizing how diligent adherence to ART can foster positive bonding and advocacy.

It must be acknowledged, of course, that some of the aforementioned recommendations might be site-specific. Despite the wide variety of stigma experiences this study details, the generalizability of the research is limited by the setting in which it took place. Although the specialty teaching hospital in which the research was conducted attracts a hybrid population, it is also a very particular urban setting. Additionally, the results of this clinic-based research may be subject to sample bias by excluding the views and experiences of clinic non-attendees, especially in light of the myriad healing choices that people with HIV/AIDS navigate. The views of people who opt not to visit a clinic or who decided not to use ART were not captured in this study, as the primary objective was to assess the lived experiences of PLWHA in relation to their use of ART. Further studies in community settings as opposed to clinics are recommended to capture data regarding people who opt out of biomedical treatment. Yet, while these limitations might restrict the generalizability of and bias of this study, they do not detract from the depth and richness of the experiences it captures and analyzes. Indeed, the study provides evidence pertaining to structural conditions (the physical layout, culture, and exigencies of clinic settings) that influence stigma and the positive outcomes that such settings engender by facilitating the formation of substitute support networks and the increased exchange of information.

Social science implications

This study implies that social science has much to offer in the study of HIV/AIDS and PLWHA. Our understanding of the disease and its effects on both individuals and society will benefit by continuing to follow the shift from an individual-based approach to one that examines the long-term, structural response to HIV by examining the social factors and cultural practices that hinder efficient prevention and treatment efforts [13]. In particular, this study further demonstrates the utility of highlighting structural and cultural factors that might undermine response measures at the individual level. It provides evidence that stigma remains a major social driver of the HIV epidemic in resource-poor settings, compromising effective illness management as well as optimal adherence to treatment.

Theoretically, stigma has generally been considered a negative factor in disease treatment; however, this study showcases that it does not have the same negative effects on everybody. Indeed, it has positive effects on some individuals and serves as a source of empowerment depending on their status in other social domains. By exploring the social dimensions of stigma, it is possible to identify the specific ways in which stigma operates within the larger socioeconomic and cultural dynamics, in particular, social contexts. Identification of how stigma affects illness management, in what circumstances it affects people, who it affects, and what other social factors synergize with it to shape illness management and lived experiences in the Ethiopian context contributes to our understanding of the ways in which social factors influence medical compliance or non-compliance. This in turn represents a contribution of medical sociology to health practices research that seeks to identify factors in the development and implementation of intervention strategies than can improve the lived experiences and illness management of PLWHA and others suffering from chronic, stigmatized diseases.

Acknowledgments

The author extends her sincere thanks and appreciation to the people living with HIV/AIDS for their participation in this study and the clinic staff for their cooperation during fieldwork. The author also wishes to express her thanks to Professors Carol Heimer, Wendy Griswold, and Celeste Watkins- Hayes at Northwestern University for their support at all stages of this research and to Elizabeth Lenaghan for reading and commenting on this work. Finally, thanks are due to the author's loving family for their unwavering support throughout this project.

References

[1] Federal Ministry of Health. *AIDS in Ethiopia: Sixth report.* Addis Ababa, Ethiopia: Ministry Health, 2006.

[2] Garbus L. *HIV/AIDS in Ethiopia: Country profile.* San Francisco, CA: AIDS Policy Research Center, University California, 2003.

[3] Federal Ministry of Health. *Ethiopian national behavioral surveillance survey BSS* [serial on the Internet], 2005.

[4] Banteyerga H, Kidanu A, Nyblade L, MacQuarrie K, Pande R. *Exploring HIV and AIDS stigma and related discrimination in Ethiopia: Causes, manifestations, consequences and coping mechanisms.* Addis Ababa: Miz-Hasab Research Center, 2003.

[5] Federal Ministry of Health. *Health and Health Related Indicators* 2005/2006. Addis Ababa, Ethiopia, 2006.

[6] World Health Organization. *Progress on global access to HIV antiretroviral therapy: An update on 3 by 5. Geneva, Switzerland*: WHO, 2005.

[7] Bernays S, Rhodes T, Terzic KJ. *"You should be grateful to have medicines": Continued dependence, altering stigma and the HIV treatment experience in Serbia. Aids Care-Psychological and Socio-Medical Aspects of AIDS/HIV* [proceedings paper]. 2010;22:14-20.

[8] Alonzo AA, Reynolds NR. Stigma, HIV and AIDS: An exploration and elaboration of a stigma trajectory. Soc Sci Med 1995;41(3):303-15.

[9] Herek GM. Thinking about AIDS and stigma: A psychologist's perspective. *J. Law Med. Ethics* 2002;30:594-607.

[10] Fife BL, Wright ER. The dimensionality of stigma: A comparison of its impact on the self of persons with HIV/AIDS and cancer. *J. Health Soc. Behav.* 2000;41(1):50-67.

[11] Mak WS, Mo PKH, Cheung RYM, Woo J, Cheung FM, Lee D. Comparative stigma of HIV/AIDS, SARS, and tuberculosis in Hong Kong. *Soc. Sci. Med.* 2006;63:1912-22.

[12] Parker R, Aggleton P. HIV and AIDS-related stigma and discrimination: A conceptual framework and implications for action. *Soc. Sci. Med.* 2003;57:13-24.

[13] Auerbach J D, Parkhurst JO, Cáceres CF. Addressing social drivers of HIV/AIDS for the long-term response: Conceptual and methodological considerations. *Glob. Publ. Health* 2011;1-17.

[14] Goffman E. Stigma: *Notes on the management of spoiled identity.* Englewood Cliffs, NJ: Prentice-Hall, 1963.

[15] Gilbert L. 'My biggest fear was that people would reject me once they knew my status . . .': Stigma as experienced by patients in an HIV/AIDS clinic in Johannesburg, South Africa. *Health Soc. Care Comm.* 2010;18(2):139-46.

[16] Holzemer WL, Uys L, Makoae L, Stewart A, Phetlhu R, Dlamini PS, et al. A conceptual model of HIV/AIDS stigma from five African countries. *J Adv Nurs* 2007;58(6):541-51.

[17] Deacon H. Towards a sustainable theory of health-related stigma: Lessons from the HIV/AIDS literature. *J. Comm. Appl. Soc. Psychol.* 2006;16:418-25.

[18] Stein J. HIV/AIDS stigma: The latest dirty secret. *Afr. J. AIDS Res.* 2003;2(2):95-101.

[19] Colbert AM, Kim KH, Sereika SM, Erlen JA. An examination of the relationships among gender, health status, social support, and HIV-related stigma. *J. Assoc. Nurs. AIDS Care* 2010;21:302-13.

[20] Castro A, Farmer P. Understanding and addressing AIDS-related stigma: From anthropological theory to clinical practice in Haiti. *Am. J. Public Health* 2005;95(1): 53-9.

[21] Wolfe WR, Weiser SD, Leiter K, Steward WT, Percy-de Korte F, Phaladze N, et al. The impact of universal access to antiretroviral therapy on HIV stigma in Botswana. *Am. J. Public Health* 2008;98(10):1865-71.

[22] Roura M, Urassa M, Busza J, Mbata D, Wringe A, Zaba B. Scaling up stigma? The effects of antiretroviral roll-out on stigma and HIV testing. Early evidence from rural Tanzania. *Sex Transm. Infect.* 2009;85(4):308-12.

[23] Campbell C, Skovdal M, Madanhire C, Mugurungi O, Gregson S, Nyamukapa C. "We, the AIDS people. . .": How antiretroviral therapy enables Zimbabweans living with HIV/AIDS to cope with stigma. *Am. J. Public Health* 2011;101(6):1004-10.

[24] Dlamini PS, Wantland D, Makoae LN, Chirwa M, Kohi TW, Greeff M, et al. HIV stigma and missed medications in HIV-positive people in five African countries. *Aids Patient Care Stds* 2009;23(5):377-87.

[25] Rintamaki LS, Davis TC, Skripkauskas S, Bennett CL, Wolf MS. Social stigma concerns and HIV medication adherence. *AIDS Patient Care Stds* 2006;20(5):359-68.

[26] Bogart LM, Wagner GJ, Galvan FH, Klein DJ. Longitudinal relationships between antiretroviral treatment adherence and discrimination due to HIV-serostatus, race, and sexual orientation among African–American men with HIV. *Ann. Behav. Med.* 2010;40:184-90.

[27] Weiser S, Wolfe W, Bangsberg D, Thior I, Gilbert P, Makhema J, et al. Barriers to antiretroviral adherence for patients living with HIV infection and AIDS in Botswana. *J. Acquir Immune Defic. Syndr.* 2003; 34(3):281-8.

[28] Gebremariam MK, Bjune GA, Frich JC. Barriers and facilitators of adherence to TB treatment in patients on concomitant TB and HIV treatment: A qualitative study. *BMC Public Health* 2010;10:651.

[29] Lopez KA, Willis DG. Descriptive Versus Interpretive Phenomenology: Their Contributions to Nursing Knowledge. *Qual Health Res.* 2004;14(5):726-35.

[30] Conrad P. The social meaning of AIDS. *Soc. Policy* 1986;17(51).

[31] Siegel K, Schrimshaw EW, Raveis VH. Accounts for non-adherence to antiviral combination therapies among older HIV-infected adults. *Psych. Health Med.* 2000;5(1):29-42.

[32] Vanable PA, Carey MP, Blair DC, Littlewood RA. Impact of HIV-related stigma on health behaviors and psychological adjustment among HIV-positive men and women. *AIDS Behav.* 2006;10:473.

[33] Zhou YR. "If you get AIDS ...you have to endure it alone": Understanding the social constructions of HIV/AIDS in China. *Soc. Sci. Med.* 2007;65(2):284-95.

[34] Carr RL, Gramling LF. Stigma: A health barrier for women with HIV/AIDS. *J. Assoc. Nurs. AIDS Care* 2004;15:30-9.

[35] Campbell C, Nair Y, Maimane S, Nicholson J. 'Dying twice': A multi-level model of the roots of AIDS stigma in two South African communities. *J. Health Psychol.* 2007;12(3):403-16.

In: Human Immunodeficiency Virus …
Editors: Hugh Klein and Joav Merrick

ISBN: 978-1-62081-293-8

Chapter VI

Condom use attitudes and HIV risk among American MSM seeking partners for unprotected sex via the internet

Hugh Klein*[*,1] and Rachel L. Kaplan[2]
[1]Kensington Research Institute, Silver Spring, Maryland
[2]Mack Center on Mental Health and Social Conflict, School of Social Welfare, University of California–Berkeley, Berkeley, California, US

Abstract

This chapter examines attitudes toward condom use in a national random sample of 332 MSM who use the Internet to seek men with whom they can engage in unprotected sex. Data collection was conducted via telephone interviews between January 2008 and May 2009. The following three research questions were addressed: 1) How do these men feel about using condoms, both ideologically and personally? 2) How do condom use attitudes relate to actual HIV risk behavior practices? 3) What factors underlie men's attitudes toward condom use? The findings indicated that men held weakly-positive attitudes toward condom use overall, but were noticeably more negative in their attitudes regarding the personal use of condoms. Condom use attitudes were related consistently and inversely to involvement in HIV risk practices. In both multivariate and structural equation analyses, men's condom-related attitudes were the single strongest factor associated with their involvement in risky sex. A number of factors were found to be correlated with more favorable attitudes toward condom use. These were: caring about potential sex partners' HIV serostatus, experiencing fewer drug-related problems, having a lower level of educational attainment, not preferring to have "wild" or "uninhibited" sex, higher self-esteem, being African American, and not perceiving great accuracy in the information that sex partners supply verbally about their HIV serostatus.

[*] Correspondence: Hugh Klein, PhD, 401 Schuyler Road, Silver Spring, Maryland 20910 United States. E-mail: hughk@aol.com (primary) and hughkhughk@yahoo.com (secondary)

Introduction

Men who have sex with men (MSM) represent one of the groups considered most at risk for the sexual transmission of HIV, at least in part due to their comparatively high risk per exposure via anal sex. The risk per exposure is estimated to be 1.00% for receptive anal sex and 0.06% for insertive anal sex as compared to 0.01-0.32% for receptive vaginal sex and 0.01-0.10% for insertive vaginal sex [1]. As condoms represent an effective method of HIV prevention, extensive efforts have been made by researchers to understand condom use attitudes in a variety of populations and to promote consistent condom use. In the United States, recent research shows that among MSM, increases in safer sex fatigue are associated with increases in the number of partners with whom they reported engaging in unprotected sex [2]. Surprisingly, there has been limited research addressing condom-related attitudes among MSM in the United States. A few studies, however, have examined condom attitudes and behavior in subpopulations of MSM, such as African American MSM [3,4], Latino MSM [5], and methamphetamine-using HIV-positive MSM [6]. These studies have shown that, among African American MSM, stronger peer condom use norms were associated with a lower frequency of risk behavior involvement [3] and lesser involvement in HIV risk behavior was associated with the perception of social norms that support condom use [4]. In a sample of Latino MSM, participants most commonly cited pleasure as the reason for a lack of condom use [5]. In a sample of methamphetamine-using HIV-positive MSM, researchers found that among men with negative attitudes about condoms, there was an association between methamphetamine use frequency and unprotected sex [6].

Although condoms are highly effective for HIV prevention when used correctly, research has shown that most individuals do not use condoms consistently [7], and others intentionally seek partners for unprotected sex. Previous research indicates a variety of factors associated with the motivation among MSM for barebacking (that is, the intentional practice of engaging in unprotected anal intercourse) [8]. These factors include the desire to: cope with psychosocial vulnerabilities [9], create intimacy with partners [9], exchange semen [10], maximize physical and/or emotional pleasure [11], and overcome social isolation [12]. Research efforts are underway to develop alternative methods of HIV prevention that are acceptable among MSM [13]. Condoms are currently the best known strategy for HIV prevention during sexual contact. Therefore, understanding the condom-related attitudes and behavior of men who seek other men for unprotected sexual contact is an important part of strategizing ways in which this subpopulation of MSM can increase safety and health by preventing HIV infection. As we previously noted, though, little has been written about condom-related attitudes among MSM, especially with regard to specific attitudes about particular aspects of condom use (e.g., perceived inconvenience, embarrassment regarding use, discomfort, etc.). Most of the published studies have reported, simply, that negative attitudes toward condoms were associated with greater involvement in risky practices [14].

Recent research has examined the use of the Internet among MSM for meeting potential sex partners, typically finding that this practice is associated with a variety of HIV risk behaviors. For example, one recent study [15] showed that 40% of MSM Internet users acknowledged engaging in unprotected anal sex. Similarly, in a study comparing self-identified barebackers and non-barebackers, barebackers were more likely to spend more time on the Internet looking for potential sex partners [16]. Furthermore, researchers have found that men who seek sex online report more unprotected sex and sexually transmitted infections compared to their peers who do not use the Internet to identify sex partners [17,18]. In a study that examined online ads and profiles on MSM-oriented unprotected sex-focused websites, the rates of advertised high-risk sexual behaviors were very high, including oral sex with ejaculation in the mouth (88.0% receptive, 77.4% insertive), anal sex with ejaculation in the anus (79.7% insertive, 69.4% receptive), multiple partner sex (77.9%), and felching (16.5%) [19]. Evidence shows increasing numbers of young MSM who meet their first sexual partner online [20]. In another sample of MSM who use the Internet, guessing the HIV serostatus of the sexual partner, as compared to checking the online profile and pre- and post-sex discussions, was associated with higher levels of unprotected anal sex [21].

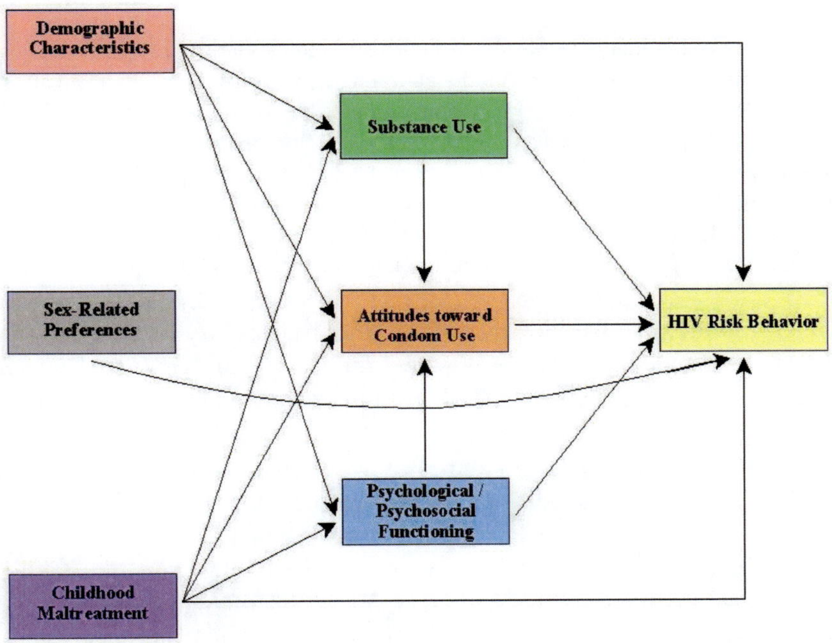

Figure 1. Conceptual model.

In the present paper, a structural approach is used to develop a better understanding of how attitudes toward condom use are related to HIV risk taking in a sample of men who use the Internet specifically to find other men with whom they can engage in unprotected sex. Based on previously published studies, the conceptual model depicted in Figure 1 was examined. In this model, attitudes toward condom use are conceptualized as an endogenous measure–that is, both as an independent variable, contributing to the understanding of men's involvement in risky behaviors, and as a dependent variable, varying based upon the effects of numerous other types of measures. As the conceptual model shows, condom-related attitudes are one of six types of influences hypothesized to affect men's HIV risk practices. The others are demographic variables (e.g., race/ethnicity, age, HIV serostatus), sex-related behavioral preferences (e.g., self-identification as a sexual "top" versus a "bottom," preferring to have sex that is "wild" or "uninhibited"), substance use/abuse, childhood maltreatment experiences, and psychological/ psychosocial functioning (e.g., depression, self-esteem, impulsivity).

To a great extent, this conceptual model owes its intellectual origins to the notion of syndemic and to Syndemics Theory. "Syndemic" refers to the tendency for multiple epidemics to co-occur and, in the process of affecting some of the same people, for the various maladies to interact with one another, with each one worsening the effects of the others [22,23]. Walkup et al [24] noted that health problems may be construed as syndemic when two or more conditions/afflictions are linked in such a manner that they interact synergistically, with each contributing to an excess burden of disease in a particular population. It is noteworthy that their work addresses the syndemic of HIV, substance abuse, and mental illness. A good example of how conditions may become syndemic is offered by Romero-Daza et al [25] in their study of sex work. The authors wrote:

> Streetwalkers' continuous exposure to violence, both as victims and as witnesses, often leaves them suffering from major emotional trauma. In the absence of adequate support services, women who have been victimized may turn to drug use in an attempt to deal with the harsh realities of their daily lives. In turn, the need for drugs, coupled with a lack of educational and employment opportunities, may lead women into prostitution. Life on the street increases women's risk for physical, emotional, and sexual abuse as well as their risk for HIV/AIDS. Exposure to traumatic experiences deepens the dependence on drugs, completing a vicious cycle of violence, substance abuse, and AIDS risk (pp. 233-234)

A number of authors, particularly during the past few years, have written about syndemics and the Syndemics Theory, as they apply it to the HIV epidemic [23,25-27], including specific mention of the applicability of the concept and theory as to men who have sex with men [27].

Using the conceptual model shown above, in the present study, we examine a population of MSM who used the Internet specifically to find partners for unprotected sex. Our focus in this paper is to examine attitudes toward condom use among men in this population. Specifically, we address the following research questions: 1) How do members of this population feel about condom use–both condom use in general and condom use as it applies to the men themselves? 2) How, if at all, do condom-related attitudes relate to men's involvement in HIV risk practices? 3) What factors are associated with having more favorable attitudes regarding condom use?

Our study

This chapter draws from data that were collected between January 2008 and May 2009 for The Bareback Project, a study funded by the National Institute on Drug Abuse. The study sample consisted of men who use the Internet specifically to find other men with whom they can engage in unprotected sex. Some of the 16 websites from which the sample of 332 men were recruited catered exclusively to unprotected sex (e.g., Bareback.com, RawLoads.com). Other websites used did not cater to unprotected sex exclusively but did make it possible for site users to identify which individuals were looking for unprotected sex (e.g., Men4SexNow.com, Squirt.org). Using the 16 websites, a national random sample of risk-seeking MSM was derived. Random selection was based on a combination of the first letter of the person's online username, his race/ethnicity (as listed in his profile), and the day of recruitment. Men of color were oversampled, to ensure good representation of men belonging to racial minority groups and to facilitate the examination of racial differences in risk behaviors and risk-related preferences. Recruitment took place seven days a week, during all hours of the day and night, varying from week to week throughout the project, to maximize the representativeness of the research sample, in recognition of the fact that different people use the Internet at different times.

Initially, men were approached for participation either via instant message or email (much more commonly via email), depending upon the website used. Potential participants were provided with a brief overview of the study and informed consent-related information, and they were given the opportunity to ask questions about the study before deciding whether or not to participate. Potential participants were also provided with a website link to the project's online home page, to offer additional information about the project and to help them feel secure in the legitimacy of the research endeavor. Interested men were scheduled for an interview soon after they expressed an interest in taking part in the study, typically within a few days. To maximize convenience for participants, interviews were conducted during all hours of the day and night, seven days a week, based on interviewer availability and participants' preferences. All of the study's interviewers were gay or lesbian, to engender credibility with the target population and to enhance participants' comfort during the interviews.

Participants completed a one-time, confidential telephone interview addressing a wide array of topics. The questionnaire that was used was developed specifically for The Bareback Project. Many parts of the survey instrument were derived from standardized scales previously used and validated by other researchers. The interview covered such subjects as: degree of "outness," perceived discrimination based on sexual orientation, general health practices, HIV testing history and serostatus, sexual practices (protected and unprotected) with partners met online and offline, risk-related preferences, risk-related hypothetical situations, substance use, drug-related problems, Internet usage, psychological and psychosocial functioning, childhood maltreatment experiences, HIV/AIDS knowledge, and some basic demographic information. The interviews lasted an average of 69 minutes (median = 63, s.d. = 20.1, range = 30–210). Participants who completed the interview were offered $35. Approval of the research protocol was given by the institutional review boards at Morgan State University (approval number 07/12-0145), where the principal investigator and one of the research assistants were affiliated, and George Mason University (approval number 5659), where the other research assistant was located.

Measures used

The principal variable of interest in this research is a 17-item scale pertaining to men's attitudes toward condom use. Individual items were scored on a five-point Likert scale, and higher scores on the scale corresponded with more conducive attitudes toward condom use. The scale was derived from the work of Brown [28] and it was found to be highly reliable (Cronbach's alpha = 0.91). Only items that were relevant to MSM and their sexual practices were used, so that the scale would be applicable to the study population.

For the second part of the analysis, examining the relationship between condom attitudes and risk practices, several *HIV risk practice measures* were examined, all using a past-30-day time frame of reference. These included: overall proportion of sex acts involving the use of condoms (a continuous measure based on responses to separate items inquiring about oral, anal, and vaginal sex), proportion of anal sex acts involving the use of condoms (a continuous measure derived from the variables just described), overall proportion of sex acts involving internal ejaculation (a continuous measure based on responses to separate items inquiring about where ejaculation occurred during oral, anal, and vaginal sex), proportion of anal sex acts involving internal ejaculation (a continuous measure derived from the items just described), having any sexual relations while under the influence of alcohol and/or other drugs (yes/no), number of male sex partners (continuous), number of times having "wild" or "uninhibited" sex (self-defined, continuous measure), and number of times having sex of any kind in a gay bath house or sex club (continuous). Men's estimated total number of lifetime sex partners was also examined (continuous).

For the third part of the analysis, focusing on identifying the factors associated with better/worse attitudes toward condom use, a variety of factors in several domains were considered. The first consisted of *demographic and background variables*. These were: age (continuous), race/ethnicity (categorical), sexual orientation (gay versus bisexual), relationship status (involved versus not involved), educational attainment (continuous), and sexual role identity (top, versatile top, versatile, versatile bottom, bottom).

The second consisted of several *HIV-related measures*. These included: HIV serostatus (positive, negative, unknown), knowing anyone currently living with HIV or AIDS (two separate yes/no measures), the number of people known who died from AIDS (continuous), preferred HIV serostatus of sex partners (positive, negative, does not matter), perceived accuracy of HIV serostatus information provided verbally by sex partners (ordinal), and perceived accuracy of online HIV serostatus information (ordinal).

The third domain pertained to men's *risk-related preferences* for sexual practices, including how rough they preferred their sex to be (continuous), how long they most liked their sexual sessions to last (continuous), how much they liked having sex in public venues (continuous), how much they liked having sex that was "wild" or "uninhibited" (continuous), and liking to have anonymous sex (yes/no).

The fourth domain pertained to *substance use/abuse* and included the following measures: currently a user of illegal drugs (yes/no), number of drug problems experienced (continuous), and total amount of illegal drug use (continuous measure of quantity × frequency of recent use, summed across nine drug types).

The final domain assessed *psychological and psychosocial functioning*. Measures examined were: self-esteem (using the Rosenberg self-esteem scale [29]; Cronbach's alpha = 0.89), impulsivity (derived from the Barratt Impulsiveness Scale [30]; Cronbach's alpha = 0.76), depression (using the CES-D [31]; Cronbach's alpha = 0.93), optimism about the future (using the Life Orientation Test–Revised [32]; Cronbach's alpha = 0.78), current life satisfaction (adapted from the Satisfaction with Life scale [33]; Cronbach's alpha = 0.83), HIV/AIDS information burnout (derived from HIV Knowledge Questionnaire [34]; Cronbach's alpha = 0.76), and childhood maltreatment experiences (separate measures for sexual abuse, physical abuse, emotional abuse, and neglect, taken from the Childhood Trauma Questionnaire [35]; Cronbach's alpha = 0.94).

Analysis

Part 1 of the analysis, focusing on identifying men's attitudes toward condom use, relied upon descriptive statistics. Part 2, examining the relationship between condom attitudes and involvement in risk practices, primarily used simple regression as the analytical strategy, as the independent variable and all but one of the dependent variables examined were continuous in nature. The one exception–whether or not the person had engaged in any recent sex while under the influence of alcohol and/or other drugs–was dichotomous, thereby making logistic regression the appropriate analytical tool.

Part 3, focusing on the factors associated with men's condom-related attitudes, was undertaken in two steps. First, bivariate relationships were assessed for each of the independent variables outlined above and condom attitudes, using the latter as the dependent variable. Whenever the independent measure was dichotomous (e.g., sexual orientation, HIV-positive serostatus), Student's t tests were used. Whenever the independent variable was continuous (e.g., educational attainment, self-esteem level), simple regression was used. Then, all items found to be related either significantly ($p<.05$) or marginally ($.15>p>.05$) to condom-related attitudes were entered into a multivariate equation, and then removed in stepwise fashion until a best fit model containing only statistically-significant measures remained.

In Part 4, the relationships depicted in Figure 2 (which were the result of the Part 2 and Part 3 analysis) were subjected to a structural equation analysis to determine whether the way the relationships depicted there are an appropriate and effective representation of the study data. SAS's PROC CALIS procedure was used to assess the overall fit of the model to the data. When we use this type of structural equation analysis, we look for several specific outcomes: (1) a goodness-of-fit index as close to 1.00 as possible, but no less than 0.90, (2) a Bentler-Bonett normed fit index value as close to 1.00 as possible, but no less than 0.90, (3) an overall chi-square value for the model that is statistically nonsignificant, preferably as far from attaining statistical significance as possible, and (4) a root mean square error approximation value as close to 0.00 as possible, but no greater than 0.05. If these conditions are met, then the relationships depicted are considered to indicate a good fit with the data.

Throughout all of the analyses, results are reported as statistically significant whenever $p<.05$.

Our findings

In total, 332 men participated in the study. They ranged in age from 18 to 72 (mean = 43.7, s.d. = 11.2, median = 43.2). Racially, the sample is a fairly close approximation of the American population, with 74.1% being Caucasian, 9.0% each being African American and Latino, 5.1% self-identifying as biracial or multiracial, 2.4% being Asian, and 0.3% being Native American. The large majority of the men (89.5%) considered themselves to be gay and almost all of the rest (10.2%) said they were bisexual. On balance, men participating in The Bareback Project were fairly well-educated. About 1 man in 7 (14.5%) had completed no more than high school; 34.3% had some college experience without earning a college degree; 28.9% had a bachelor's degree; and 22.3% were educated beyond the bachelor's level.

Slightly more than one-half of the men (59.0%) reported being HIV-positive; most of the rest (38.6%) were HIV-negative.

Attitudes toward condom use

Overall, men's attitudes toward condom use were rather ambivalent, averaging 2.96 on a 1–5 scale (see Table 1). On the positive side, most study participants felt that men should not be embarrassed to suggest a condom (93.0%), that using a condom was not a reason for feeling embarrassment (83.0%), and that they would not object if one of their partners asked them to use a condom (61.8%).

Table 1. Attitudes toward Condom Use

Attitude Item	Percentage Disagreeing	Percentage Neutral	Percentage Agreeing
* In your opinion, condoms are too much trouble.	31.8	19.4	48.8
Condoms are unreliable.	16.7	18.8	64.5
* Condoms are pleasant to use	74.6	15.2	10.3
There is no reason why a man should be embarrassed to suggest a condom.	3.3	3.6	93.0
* You think that proper use of condoms can enhance sexual pleasure.	63.9	16.7	19.4
Many people make using condoms an erotic part of foreplay.	35.5	27.6	37.0
* You just don't like the idea of using condoms.	65.5	13.0	21.5
* You think condoms look ridiculous.	18.2	18.2	63.6
Condoms are inconvenient.	55.2	14.8	30.0
You see no reason to be embarrassed by the use of condoms.	8.2	8.8	83.0
* Putting a condom on an erect penis can be a real sexual turn-on.	63.9	15.2	20.9
* Condoms are uncomfortable.	57.3	13.9	28.8
* Using a condom makes sex unenjoyable.	47.0	18.5	34.5
*You would avoid using condoms if at all possible.	70.6	9.7	19.7
Putting on a condom is an interruption of foreplay.	50.6	16.1	33.3
* There is no way that using a condom can be pleasant.	25.5	18.2	56.4
* You would have no objection if your partner suggested that you use a condom.	29.1	9.1	61.8

* Attitude toward personal condom use.

But on the negative side, most study participants felt that condoms were unreliable (64.5%), that they were not pleasant to use (74.6%), that their use could not enhance sexual pleasure (63.9%), that they looked ridiculous (63.6%), and that putting on a condom was a sexual turn-off (63.9%).

Nearly two-thirds of the men studied said that they simply do not like the idea of using condoms (65.5%) and even more of the men said that they would avoid using condoms if at all possible (70.6%).

As Table 1 also shows, if a differentiation is made between men's attitudes toward condom use in general (that is, condom use as a concept, not applied to their specific behaviors) and their attitudes toward using condoms themselves (that is, attitudes toward personal condom use), a rather different picture emerges. Whereas men's attitudes toward condom use in general were positive overall (mean score = 3.38), their attitudes toward personal condom use were noticeably more negative (mean score = 2.73).

Table 2. Attitudes toward Condom Use and Involvement in Risky Sex

Risk Behavior Measure	Overall Condom-Related Attitudes	Attitudes toward Personal Condom Use
% of protected sex acts	*p*<.0001	*p*=.0005
% of protected anal sex	*p*<.0001	*p*<.0001
% of sex acts with internal ejaculation	*p*<.0001	*p*=.0014
% of anal sex acts with internal ejaculation	*p*<.0001	*p*=.0004
had any sex while "under the influence"	*p*=.0003	*p*=.0009
number of recent sex partners	*p*<.0001	*p*<.0001
number of lifetime sex partners	*p*<.0001	*p*=.0011
number of times recently having "wild" or "uninhibited" sex	*p*=.0005	*p*=.0006
number of times recently having sex in a gay bath house or a sex club	*p*=.0356	*p*=.0334

Condom-related attitudes and behavioral risk

As expected, men's attitudes toward condom use were related closely to their involvement in sexual risk practices (see Table 2). This was true for the global measure of condom-related attitudes and for the component measure of attitudes toward personal condom use. In every instance, more favorable attitudes toward condom use were associated with lesser involvement in risky sex. This was true for the overall proportion of all sex acts involving the use of condoms (p<.0001), the proportion of anal sex acts involving the use of condoms (p<.0001), the proportion of all sex acts involving internal ejaculation (p<.0001), the proportion of anal sex acts involving internal ejaculation (p<.0001), the likelihood that the person recently had engaged in any sex acts while under the influence of alcohol and/or other drugs (p=.0003), the number of sex partners that the person reported having had recently and during his lifetime (both p<.0001), the number of times recently having engaged in sex adjudged by the man himself to be "wild" or "uninhibited" (p=.0005), and the number of times recently having had sex in a place like a gay bath house or a sex club (p=.036).

When examined via multivariate analysis, condom-related attitudes are the single strongest factor associated with men's involvement in risky sex. One specific example demonstrating this is presented in Figure 2, where the outcome measure is the proportion of all sex acts involving the use of condoms. Six variables were found to be related uniquely to the equation. First, knowing people who are currently living with AIDS was associated with greater condom use when compared to people who knew no one currently living with AIDS (ß=.11, p=.034). Coinciding with this, knowing people who died from AIDS was associated with protecting oneself with condoms (ß=.12, p=.032). Third, men who were HIV-positive used condoms less than one-half as much as their HIV-negative and serostatus-unknown counterparts (ß=.17, p=.002). Fourth, Caucasian men engaged in about one-third as much protected sex as their nonwhite counterparts (ß=.17, p=.002). Fifth, the more confident men were in the truthfulness of HIV serostatus information supplied to them by their sex partners, the less they tended to use condoms (ß=.15, p=.006). Finally, the more positive men's attitudes toward using condoms were, the more they tended to practice protected sex (ß=.29, p<.0001). Together, these items explained 23.8% of the total variance.

Factors associated with condom-related attitudes

As Figure 2 shows, seven items contributed uniquely to the overall understanding of men's attitudes toward condom use once the effects of the other measures were taken into account. The first factor was race/ethnicity. African American men had more favorable attitudes toward condom use overall than their counterparts of other racial groups did (ß=.13, p=.008). The second factor was educational attainment, with higher education tending to be linked with greater opposition to condom use (ß=.13, p=.010). The third factor was not caring about potential sex partners' HIV serostatus. Men who said that they did not care about the HIV serostatus of potential sex partners had more negative attitudes toward condom use than did men who specifically wanted their partners to be HIV-positive or HIV-negative (ß=.15, p=.004). The fourth contributing measure was the preference for "wild" or "uninhibited" sex. The more that men wanted their sex to be "wild" or "uninhibited," the more negative their attitudes toward condoms were (ß=.24, p<.0001). The fifth factor was the number of drug problems that men experienced, with a greater number of drug-related problems (i.e., abuse/dependency symptoms) being associated with more negative attitudes toward condom use (ß=.13, p=.009). The sixth measure retained in the multivariate equation was the perceived accuracy of information provided by sex partners about their HIV serostatus. The more that men believed in the accuracy of what their sex partners told them about their HIV serostatus, the less favorably disposed they tended to be regarding condom use (ß=.15, p=.004). Finally, level of self-esteem was found to be associated with men's attitudes toward condom use, with better self-esteem corresponding to more favorable condom-related attitudes (ß=.17, p=.001). Together, in the multivariate analysis, these items explained 21.9% of the total variance.

The overall role of condom-related attitudes

Figure 2 portrays the specific role played by men's attitudes toward condom use when it comes to their involvement in protected sex. The structural equation analysis revealed that this way of depicting the data is an excellent representation of the interrelationships amongst the variables. The goodness-of-fit index for this model is 0.995, which is supported by the Bentler-Bonett normed fit index value of 0.977, indicating a strong overall "fit" for the data. The model's chi-square value is 9.52 (10df), which is not statistically significant (p=.484) and does not approach attaining statistical significance. Finally, the root mean square error approximation has a value of 0.000.

Discussion and conclusion

As with any research study, the present study has a few potential limitations. First, the response/participation rate was low (<10%), which could raise concern of selection bias and, therefore, the representativeness of the sample. Although it is difficult to be certain that the men who participated represent the men who did not, there is compelling evidence to suggest that differences between the two groups are minimal. Before The Bareback Project was implemented, the principal investigator conducted a large-scale content analysis with a random national sample of one of the main websites used by men to meet other men seeking unprotected sex partners [19,36,37]. The demographic composition of that sample and the one obtained in The Bareback Project closely match one another in terms of age representation, racial group composition, sexual orientation, and rural/suburban/urban location of residence. The two samples also resemble one another closely in terms of the types of sexual practices that men sought. The similarity of the two samples suggests that men who chose to participate in the present study represent those who did not, in terms of identifiable characteristics that are likely to be the best indicators of selection bias. Despite these similarities, the participation rate remains on the low side and thus represents a potential limitation for generalizability.

Second, as with most research data on sexual behaviors, the data in this study are based on uncorroborated self-reports. Therefore, it is unknown whether participants underreported or overreported their involvement in risky behaviors. The self-reported data probably can be trusted, however, as noted by other authors of previous studies with similar populations [38]. This is particularly relevant for self-reported measures that involve relatively small occurrences (e.g., number of times having a particular kind of sex during the previous 30 days), which characterize the substantial majority of the data collected in this study [39]. Other researchers have also commented favorably on the reliability of self-reported information in their studies regarding topics such as condom use [40].

A third potential limitation is the possibility of recall bias. For most of the measures used, respondents were asked about their beliefs, attitudes, and behaviors during the past 30 days. This time frame was chosen specifically: 1) to incorporate a large enough time frame in order to facilitate meaningful variability from person to person, and 2) to minimize recall bias. Although the authors cannot determine the exact extent to which recall bias affected the data, other researchers who have used similar measures have reported that recall bias is sufficiently minimal and that its impact upon study findings is likely to be negligible [41]. This seems to be especially true when the recall period is small [42,43], as was the case for most of the main measures used in the present study.

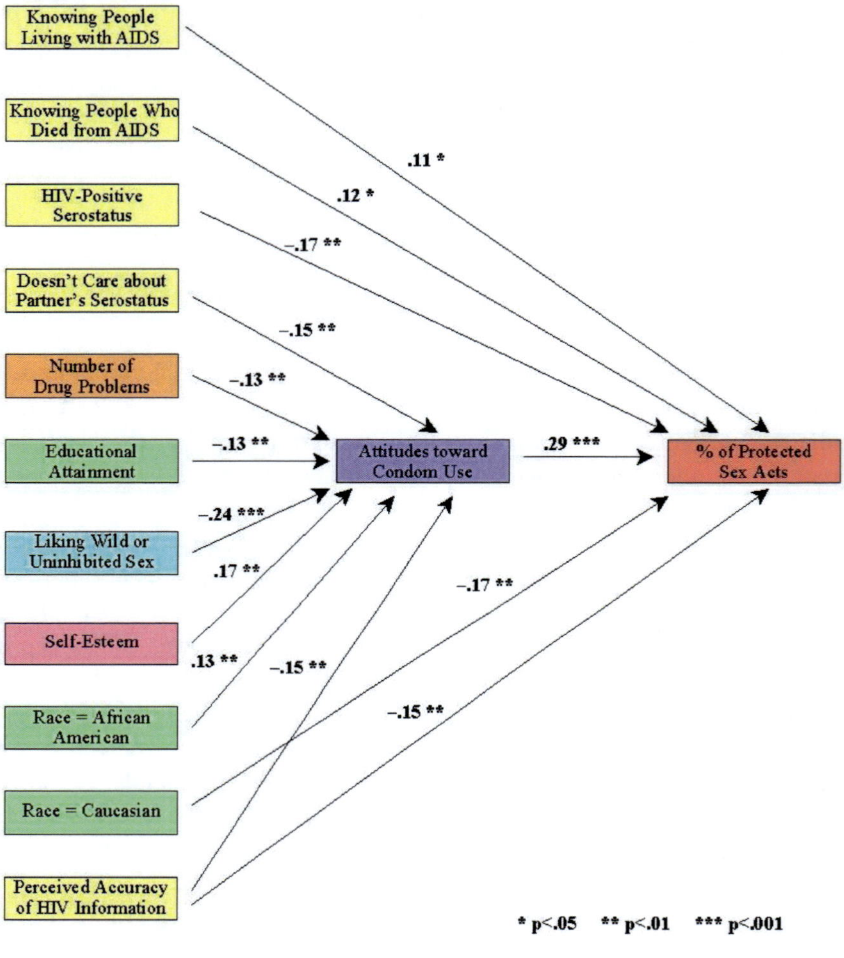

Figure 2. Condom-related attitudes and protected sex.

Despite these potential limitations, the present authors believe that the current study has much to offer. As hypothesized, condom-related attitudes were associated (consistently and inversely) with men's sexual risk practices. They were, in fact, the single strongest factor related to HIV risk identified in the structural equation model depicted in Figure 2. Reducing HIV risk in this population will depend heavily on finding ways to change how men feel about using condoms. The data indicate an important difference between men's attitudes about condoms in general and their attitudes about using them personally. Although men in the sample had weakly-positive attitudes about condoms overall, their attitudes about using condoms themselves were considerably more negative. In other words, the men were not opposed to condoms ideologically; they simply preferred not to use condoms themselves.

Thus, intervention strategies must consider the question of how to make condoms more appealing and less unpleasant to men who prefer intentional condomless sex. Previous research suggests that highlighting the sexual/sensory aspects of condoms and eroticizing safer sex might help increase condom use among MSM [7]. Indeed, when asked in the present study how they felt about the statement, "Many people make using condoms an erotic part of foreplay," men's responses were very divided (see Table 1), suggesting the possibility of making inroads in this area. Specific strategies to eroticize safer sex for members of this target population need to be developed, implemented, and subsequently tested for effectiveness. A number of community-based HIV prevention, education, and intervention programs around the United States have offered workshops about eroticizing safer sex, in an effort to teach members of the MSM community about specific strategies that can be undertaken to make condom use and other safer sex strategies more palatable. Programs such as those offered by Gay Men's Health Crisis in New York City [44], the Howard Brown Health Center in Chicago, and Project ARK in St. Louis are to be applauded, as are community-specific approaches such as AIDS Project Los Angeles' Red Circle Project (targeting safer sex among Native Americans) and Bockting, Rosser, and Scheltema's [45] program targeting safer sex among transgendered persons. Likewise, in recent years, websites dedicated to promoting erotic safer sex have begun to appear on the Internet, and we believe that they offer great promise in combating HIV risk-taking among MSM. An excellent example of this may be found on the Washington, DC-based group's DCFukit website, at www.dcfukit.org. Finding innovative ways to eroticize safer sex may be an important approach to changing how MSM think about condom use, and that, in turn, is likely to be an effective way of reducing their involvement in risky sexual practices.

One approach to accomplishing this may be to develop Internet-based prevention and intervention programs targeting the MSM community, as recent evidence has suggested that this approach may be effective in decreasing risk in this population. For example, Bowen and colleagues [46,47] tested the feasibility, acceptability, and efficacy of an Internet-based HIV prevention intervention targeting MSM in rural communities. Their preliminary findings indicated community support for such an intervention, with MSM in the study reporting reduced anal sex and increased condom usage. Likewise, another Internet-based prevention intervention among MSM demonstrated reductions in sexual contact with partners who were HIV-positive or HIV-serostatus-unknown [48]. Internet-based prevention/intervention approaches may be particularly apropos with populations similar to that involved in the present study because these men were using the Internet actively to find partners for unsafe sex.

The present study also identified several specific factors that were associated with men's attitudes toward condom use. We wish to discuss the implications of some of these findings. First, we discovered that men who said that they did not care whether their sex partners were HIV-positive or HIV-negative had more negative attitudes toward condom use overall than their counterparts who did care about their sex partners' HIV serostatus. In other research as well, a partner's indication of HIV serostatus has been shown to be linked to condom use attitudes and behaviors among MSM [5,49]. Intervention programs working with MSM need to emphasize the importance of considering one's partners' HIV serostatus as one makes decisions regarding the types of sexual behaviors in which one is/not willing to engage. Intervention messages need to emphasize the importance of considering condom use and other safer sex strategies for men who engage in sex with serodiscordant partners.

Along the same lines, the present study found that, the more accurate men perceived HIV information supplied by would-be sex partners to be, the more negative their condom-related attitudes tended to be. This finding suggests that men who ask their partners about their HIV serostatus prior to having sex are apt to rely upon that information, supplanting it for their general feelings about using condoms. If their partners tell them that they are HIV-negative, then our findings suggest that the men accept this verbal information and act accordingly. Although we believe that it is important to discuss sexual partners' HIV serostatus, this strategy does not ensure protection from HIV transmission. HIV prevention strategies targeting MSM should, therefore, emphasize the importance of making decisions on the basis of personal safety and protection without relying primarily upon a partner's word, especially if that partner is not well known by the individual in question.

This study also found that attitudes toward condom use were more positive among African American men than they were among men belonging to other racial/ethnic groups. This finding, coupled with the lower overall rates of condom use practiced by Caucasian men (see Figure 2), suggests a need to target Caucasian men in future prevention, education, and risk reduction intervention efforts. A number of published studies have reported on racial differences in HIV risk-taking among MSM [50–52], leading some authors to advocate culturally-specific targeted interventions. Our own research findings suggest a need to target Caucasian MSM, particularly those using the Internet to identify partners for unprotected sex, and to develop strategies that can be effective at modifying how these men feel about using condoms.

In conclusion, the present study found that attitudes toward condom use among MSM seeking partners for unprotected sex via the Internet are the single strongest factor associated with men's involvement in risky sex. HIV risk reduction efforts need to find ways to change the way that men feel about using condoms. They need to change the prevalent notions that condoms are unpleasant to use, that they reduce sexual pleasure, that they interrupt foreplay, and that putting them on a sex partner cannot be an erotic act–all notions that were commonplace in the men participating in this study. It is important to bear in mind that condom use attitudes do not exist or develop in isolation. The factors that help shape them (which the present study's findings suggest may be race/ethnicity, caring about sex partners' HIV serostatus, educational attainment, substance use/abuse problems, and level of self-esteem) can lead researchers toward successful prevention intervention strategies.

Social science implications

Sexual behavior and sexual risk are social and/or interpersonal by nature and cannot be examined in a contextual vacuum. Although MSM were asked individually about their sexual behaviors and attitudes, sexual behaviors themselves take place in a complex social environment. Public health strategies can appear to be at odds with an individual's choices when making personal decisions about sexual behavior. Social scientists strive to understand the social determinants of health in an effort to mitigate the impact of HIV/AIDS.

However, the importance of psychosocial functioning can, inadvertently, become secondary to disease prevention. Social scientists must seek ways to balance individuals' sexual and psychosocial needs with the larger public's health and safety. Understanding condom use attitudes and other psychosocial measures of functioning simultaneously can improve our ability to enhance individual-level and societal-level health and to address the needs of individuals more adequately. Condom use attitudes can offer clues about individuals' choices according to their social, emotional, psychological, and sexual needs. These ways of examining risk behavior and HIV transmission prevention are not applicable exclusively to MSM seeking unprotected anal intercourse (UAI). Rather, they apply across populations and are particularly relevant for discussions about decision-making processes and models such as Empowerment Theory, the Theory of Reasoned Action, and the Health Belief Model. For MSM seeking UAI, the perceived benefits of having UAI outweigh the perceived risks.

Actively seeking unprotected sex indicates a tipping of the risk / benefit scales in favor of more risk, according to health researchers and prevention specialists [53]. However, 'safe' and 'risk' are subjective terms that are defined relatively, according to individuals' needs, desires, and preferences. As social scientists, our goal is not to pathologize behaviors, such as actively seeking unprotected sex, as was the focus of this study of MSM. Instead, our efforts should include psychosocial factors and the social determinants of health that correlate with condom use and attitudes toward using condoms. Failing to do so would be a failure to understand individuals and groups comprehensively, particularly from a social science perspective on behavior that is social and/or interpersonal in nature. The findings of this study support the Health Belief Model in that MSM in the sample held beliefs about condom use that directly corresponded to their sexual risk practices. As noted, in order to promote health by reducing HIV transmission in this high-risk population, it is essential for men to change the way they view personal condom use. This, however, must be approached within the broader context of an individual's needs and psychosocial health.

Acknowledgments

This research was supported by a grant from the National Institute on Drug Abuse (5R24DA019805). The authors wish to acknowledge, with gratitude, the contributions made to this study's data collection and data entry/cleaning functions by Thomas P. Lambing.

References

[1] Levy JA. *HIV and the pathogenesis of AIDS,* 3rd ed. Washington, DC: ASM Press, 2007.

[2] Ostrow DG, Silverberg MJ, Cook RL, Chmiel JS, Johnson L, Li X, Jacobson LP. Prospective study of attitudinal and relationship predictors of sexual risk in the Multicenter AIDS Cohort Study. *AIDS Behav.* 2008;12:127-38.

[3] Bakeman R, Peterson JL, Community Intervention Trial for Youth Study Team. Do beliefs about HIV treatments affect peer norms and risky sexual behaviour among African-American men who have sex with men? *Int. J. STD AIDS* 2007;18:105-8.

[4] Peterson JL, Rothenberg R, Kraft JM, Beeker C, Trotter R. Perceived condom norms and HIV risks among social and sexual networks of young African American men who have sex with men. *Health Educ. Res.* 2009;24:119-27.

[5] Carballo-Diéguez A, Miner M, Dolezal C, Rosser BR, Jacoby S. Sexual negotiation, HIV-status disclosure, and sexual risk behavior among Latino men who use the Internet to seek sex with other men. *Arch. Sex Behav.* 2006;35:473-81.

[6] Nakamura N, Mausbach BT, Ulibarri MD, Semple SJ, Patterson TL. Methamphetamine use, attitudes about condoms, and sexual risk behavior among HIV positive men who have sex with men. *Arch. Sex Behav.* 2011;40:267-72.

[7] Scott-Sheldon LA, Marsh KL, Johnson BT, Glasford DE. Condoms + pleasure = safer sex? A missing addend in the safer sex message. *AIDS Care* 2006;18:750-4.

[8] Neville S, Adams J. Condom use in men who have sex with men: A literature review. *Contemp. Nurse* 2009;33:130-9.

[9] Bauermeister JA, Carballo-Diéguez A, Ventuneac A, Dolezal C. Assessing motivations to engage in intentional condomless anal intercourse in HIV risk contexts ("Bareback Sex") among men who have sex with men. *AIDS Educ. Prev.* 2009:21:156-68.

[10] Holmes D, Warner D. The anatomy of a forbidden desire: men, penetration and semen exchange. *Nurs. Inq.* 2005;12:10-20.

[11] Balán IC, Carballo-Diéguez A, Ventuneac A, Remien RH. Intentional condomless anal intercourse among Latino MSM who meet sexual partners on the Internet. *AIDS Educ. Prev.* 2009;21:14-24.

[12] 12. Carballo-Diéguez A, Bauermeister J. "Barebacking": intentional condomless anal sex in HIV-risk contexts. Reasons for and against it. *J. Homosex* 2004;47:1-16.

[13] Nodin N, Carballo-Diéguez A, Ventuneac AM, Balan IC, Remien R. Knowledge and acceptability of alternative HIV prevention bio-medical products among MSM who bareback. *AIDS Care* 2008;20:106-15.

[14] Whittier DK, St. Lawrence J, Seeley S. Sexual risk behavior of men who have sex with men: Comparison of behavior at home and at a gay resort. *Arch. Sex Behav.* 2005;34:95-102.

[15] Berg RC. Barebacking among MSM Internet users. *AIDS Behav.* 2008;12:822-33.

[16] Grov C, DeBusk JA, Bimbi DS, Golub SA, Nanin JE, Parsons JT. Barebacking, the Internet, and harm reduction: an intercept survey with gay and bisexual men in Los Angeles and New York City. *AIDS Behav.* 2007;11:527-36.

[17] Liau A, Millett G, Marks G. Meta-analytic examination of online sex-seeking and sexual risk behavior among men who have sex with men. *Sex Transm. Dis.* 2006;33:576-84.

[18] McKirnan D, Houston E, Tolou-Shams M. Is the web the culprit? Cognitive escape and Internet sexual risk among gay and bisexual men. *AIDS Behav.* 2007;11:151-60.

[19] Klein H. HIV risk practices sought by men who have sex with other men, and who use Internet websites to identify potential sexual partners. *Sex Health* 2008;5:243-50.

[20] Bolding G, Davis M, Hart G, Sherr L, Elford J. Where young MSM meet their first sexual partner: The role of the Internet. *AIDS Behav.* 2007;11:522-6.

[21] Horvath KJ, Nygaard K, Rosser BRS. Ascertaining partner HIV status and its association with sexual risk behavior among Internet-using men who have sex with men. *AIDS Behav.* 2010;14:1376-83.

[22] Singer M. *Introduction to syndemics: A systems approach to public and community health.* San Francisco, CA: Jossey-Bass, 2009.

[23] Singer MC, Erickson PI, Badiane L, Diaz R, Ortiz D, Abraham T, Nicolaysen AM. Syndemics, sex and the city: Understanding sexually transmitted diseases in social and cultural context. *Soc. Sci. Med.* 2006;63:2010-21.

[24] Walkup J, Blank MB, Gonzales JS, Safren S, Schwartz R, Brown L, Wilson I, Knowlton A, Lombard F, Grossman C, Lyda K, Schumacher JE. The impact of mental

health and substance abuse factors on HIV prevention and treatment. *J. Acquir Immune Defic. Syndr.* 2008;47:S15-9.

[25] Romero-Daza N, Weeks M, Singer M. "Nobody gives a damn if I live or die": Violence, drugs, and street-level prostitution in inner-city Hartford, Connecticut. *Med. Anthropol.* 2003;22:233-59.

[26] Gielen AC, Ghandour RM, Burke JG, Mahoney P, McDonnell KA, O'Campo P. HIV/AIDS and intimate partner violence: Intersecting women's health issues in the United States. *Trauma Violence Abuse* 2007;8:178-98.

[27] Mustanski B, Garofalo R, Herrick A, Donenberg G. Psychosocial health problems increase risk for HIV among urban young men who have sex with men: Preliminary evidence of a syndemic in need of attention. *Ann. Behav. Med.* 2007;34:37-45.

[28] Brown IS. Development of a scale to measure attitude toward the condom as a method of birth control. *J. Sex Res.* 1984;20:255-63.

[29] Rosenberg M. *Society and the adolescent self-image*. Princeton, NJ: Princeton University Press, 1965.

[30] Von Diemen L, Szobot CM, Kessler F, Pechansky F. Adaptation and construction of the Barratt Impulsiveness Scale BIS 11 to Brazilian Portuguese for use in adolescents. *Rev. Bras. Psiquiatr* 2007;29:153-6.

[31] Radloff LS. The CES-D scale: A self-report depression scale for research in the general population. *Appl. Psychol. Meas* 1977;1:385-401.

[32] Scheier MF, Carver CS. Optimism, coping, and health: Assessment and implications of generalized outcome expectancies. *Health Psychol.* 1985;4:219-47.

[33] Diener E, Emmons RA, Larsen RJ, Griffin S. The satisfaction with life scale. *J. Pers. Assess,* 1985;49:71-5.

[34] Carey MP, Morrison-Beedy D, Johnson B. The HIV-Knowledge Questionnaire: Development and evaluation of a reliable, valid, and practical self-administered questionnaire. *AIDS Behav.* 1997;1:61-74.

[35] Bernstein DP, Fink L. Childhood Trauma Questionnaire: A retrospective self-report manual. San Antonio, TX: *Psychological Corporation,* 1998.

[36] Klein H. Differences in HIV risk practices sought by self-identified gay and bisexual men who use Internet websites to identify potential sexual partners. *J. Bisex* 2008;9:125-40.

[37] Klein H. Sexual orientation, drug use preference during sex, and HIV risk practices and preferences among men who specifically seek unprotected sex partners via the Internet. *Int. J. Environ. Res. Publ. Health* 2009;6:1620-35.

[38] Schrimshaw EW, Rosario M, Meyer-Bahlburg HFL, Scharf-Matlick AA. Test-retest reliability of self-reported sexual behavior, sexual orientation, and psychosexual milestones among gay, lesbian, and bisexual youths. *Arch. Sex Behav.* 2006;35:225-34.

[39] Bogart LM, Walt LC, Pavlovic JD, Ober AJ, Brown N, Kalichman SC. Cognitive strategies affecting recall of sexual behavior among high-risk men and women. *Health Psychol.* 2007;26:787-93.

[40] Morisky DE, Ang A, Sneed CD. Validating the effects of social desirability on self-reported condom use behavior among commercial sex workers. *AIDS Educ. Prev.* 2002;14:351-60.

[41] Kauth MR, St. Lawrence JS, Kelly JA. Reliability of retrospective assessments of sexual HIV risk behavior: A comparison of biweekly, three-month, and twelve-month self-reports. *AIDS Educ. Prev.* 1991;3:207-14.

[42] Fenton KA, Johnson AM, McManus S, Erens B. Measuring sexual behaviour: Methodological challenges in survey research. *Sex Transm. Infect.* 2001;77:84-92.

[43] Weir SS, Roddy RE, Zekeng L, Ryan KA. Association between condom use and HIV infection: A randomised study of self reported condom use measures. *J. Epidemiol. Community Health,*1999;53:417-22.

[44] Palacios-Jimenez L, Shernoff M. *Facilitator's guide to eroticizing safer sex: A psychoeducational workshop approach to safer sex education.* New York: Gay Men's Health Crisis, 1986.

[45] Bockting WO, Rosser BRS, Scheltema K. Transgender HIV prevention: Implementation and evaluation of a workshop. *Health Educ. Res.* 1999;14:177-83.

[46] Bowen AM, Horvath K, Williams ML. A randomized control trial of Internet-delivered HIV prevention targeting rural MSM. *Health Educ. Res.* 2007;22:120-7.

[47] Bowen AM, Williams ML, Daniel CM, Clayton S. Internet based HIV prevention research targeting rural MSM: Feasibility, acceptability, and preliminary efficacy. *J. Behav. Med.* 2008;31:463-77.

[48] Carpenter KM, Stoner SA, Mikko AN, Dhanak LP, Parsons JT. Efficacy of a web-based intervention to reduce sexual risk in men who have sex with men. *AIDS Behav.* 2010;14:549-57.

[49] Horvath KJ, Oakes JM, Rosser BR. Sexual negotiation and HIV serodisclosure among men who have sex with men with their online and offline partners. *J. Urban Health* 2008;85:744-58.

[50] Millett GA, Flores SA, Peterson JL, Bakeman R. Explaining disparities in HIV infection among black and white men who have sex with men: A meta-analysis of HIV risk behaviors. *AIDS* 2007;21:2083-91.

[51] Mutchler MG, Bogart LM, Elliott MN, McKay T, Suttorp MJ, Schuster MA. Psychosocial correlates of unprotected sex without disclosure of HIV-positivity among African-American, Latino, and White men who have sex with men and women. *Arch. Sex Behav* 2008;37:736-47.

[52] Rhodes SD, Yee LJ, Hergenrather KC. A community-based rapid assessment of HIV behavioural risk disparities within a large sample of gay men in southeastern USA: A comparison of African American, Latino, and white men. *AIDS Care* 2006;18:1018-24.

[53] Adam PC, Murphy DA, de Wit JB. When do online sexual fantasies become reality? The contribution of erotic chatting via the Internet to sexual risk-taking in gay and other men who have sex with men. *Health Educ. Res.* 2011;26:506-15.

In: Human Immunodeficiency Virus ...
Editors: Hugh Klein and Joav Merrick
ISBN: 978-1-62081-293-8

Chapter VII

Beyond sexual partnerships: The lack of condom use during vaginal sex with primary partners

Lara DePadilla, Kirk W. Elifson and Claire E. Sterk*
Department of Behavioral Sciences and Health Education, Rollins School of Public Health, Emory University, Atlanta, Georgia, US

Abstract

The focus of this chapter is to identify independent correlates of the lack of condom use when engaging in vaginal sex with primary partners among HIV-negative African American adults. The conceptual model includes proximal as well as more distal domains. Cross-sectional data were collected between May 2009 and August 2011. Recruitment involved active and passive recruitment strategies. Computer-assisted, individual interviews were conducted with 1,050 African American adults. Multivariate logistic regression was used to identify independent predictors of a lack of condom use with primary partners in the past 30 days. In multivariate analysis, being older than 35, being partnered, perceiving having a primary partner as important, and ever having been homeless were associated positively with the odds of a lack of condom use during vaginal sex with primary partners in the past 30 days. On the other hand, reporting more than one primary partner in the past 30 days, having health insurance during the past 12 months, and perceived neighborhood social cohesion were negatively associated. These findings highlight the need for HIV risk-reduction prevention and intervention efforts that consider distal as well as proximal domains. Such a perspective allows for a broader sociological inquiry into health disparities that moves beyond epidemiological factors that commonly guide public health research.

Introduction

African Americans, specifically those belonging to the lower socioeconomic strata and living in disadvantaged urban neighborhoods, have been impacted disproportionately by HIV [1]. In 2009, African Americans comprised 14% of the United States population, but 44% of new HIV infections occurred among them [2]. Between 2005 and 2008, African Americans experienced the largest increase in rate of HIV diagnoses as compared to members of other racial groups [2]. In addition, African Americans were found to have the highest lifetime risk for a diagnosis of HIV infection of all racial/ethnic groups. Specifically, the rate among African Americans was one in 22 as compared to a rate of one in 170 among whites, and one in 52 among Hispanics/Latinos [3]. These data also show that, by region in the U.S., African Americans accounted for the majority of HIV cases in the South (55.7%) [3].

Since the 1990s, social scientists have called for a "syndemic" approach to the HIV epidemic and associated disparities [4-7]. In the public health community, the increasing need for recognizing such an approach is reflected in an emerging body of literature on multi-level approaches to the HIV/AIDS epidemic, including an emphasis on the social determinants of health and health disparities [8-10]. By placing individual behaviors in the larger context of social inequality, poverty, unequal access to health care, uneven criminal justice involvement, and residence in crumbling neighborhoods with limited social capital, tailored prevention and intervention efforts may be more likely to be effective in curtailing the devastating impact of the HIV/AIDS epidemic on African Americans. As one of its main goals, the National HIV/AIDS Strategy calls for prioritizing the reduction of HIV-related health disparities [11]. Given that condom use as a safer sex strategy remains one of the most effective risk-reduction strategies among African Americans, especially in the U.S. South where much of the epidemic is driven by heterosexual transmission [3], we focus on condom use during vaginal sex with primary partners. Specifically, we aim to gain a better understanding of distal and proximal factors that influence the use of condoms during vaginal sex with primary partners. Examples of proximal factors include relationships and sexual partnerships and in the more distal domain, socioeconomic status and neighborhood social capital.

Partner type and condom use

The way in which a person categorizes a sex partner likely will determine condom use behavior. In this inquiry, we limit the focus to male condoms because the use of female condoms is relatively low in the United States [12]. Among women, researchers have found condom use with new or casual partners to be more common than condom use with regular partners [13]. In addition, study findings show condom use to be least consistent with primary partners and explanations given for this include the notion that a primary partnership, beyond a sexual engagement, also involves emotional connectedness and trust [14, 15]. The identification of the nature of a partner type (e.g., primary and casual) typically is left to study participants. Consequently, researchers as well as prevention and intervention experts may be applying definitions that do not capture everyday complexities of primary and casual partnerships, with the latter including transactional sex for which one partner is paid and the other pays. Having sex with a primary partner has been associated with a decrease in the odds of protected vaginal sex among women [16,17], while having sex with a casual partner has been associated with an increased likelihood of condom use among women as well as men [18]. Among the barriers to condom use identified in the context of sex with primary partners are the perceived distraction from sexual intimacy and a possible reduction of sexual pleasure, its association with distrust in a partner and the assumption of unfaithfulness, and inadequate communication and negotiation skills [14,19,20]. Foregoing condom use with a primary partner may serve as a means of establishing trust [21]. When examining gender, some researchers found that women generally are more communicative about condom use and safer sex than men [22,23], although others found no gender differences [24,25].

Much of the research on condom use and sex partner type has focused on at-risk individuals, which include vulnerable African American men and women [26] who live in a social context characterized by distress that is triggered by negative social conditions such as poverty, easy access to alcohol and other drugs, and limited social cohesion. Several researchers found such macro-level factors to lead to partner concurrency [27,28]. Partner concurrency refers to having multiple sex partners during the same time period, possibly including primary and non-primary partners. Partner concurrency has been associated with a higher number of unprotected vaginal sex acts with all types of sex partners, including primary and non-primary partners alike, but not specifically with primary partners [29]. The impact of having more than one partner and how the partners are categorized may be important to consider when examining partner types and condom use.

Socioeconomic status, social capital and condom use

Recognizing the influence of the larger socioeconomic context on condom use, it seems important to consider factors such as employment, income, and economic stability when exploring reasons for using or not using condoms. Economic hardship has been shown to have a negative association with condom use in a national sample of young adults [30]. Perhaps as an example of extreme economic difficulties, being homeless has been found to be associated with unprotected sex among women as their homeless status resulted in more immediate challenges for daily survival and might overshadow the long-term HIV risk due to unprotected sex [17]. Finally, being in an economically motivated sexual relationship was associated with reduced condom use among African American women [31]. The authors hypothesize that this is because the women's limited financial and material resources results in a reliance on sex partners and cultural norms in the women's social and sexual networks may be more accepting of economically motivated sexual relationships. It may also be that women in such relationships who do not use condoms seek to emulate primary relationships where sexual intimacy is driven by mutual trust as opposed to financial support [14].

Social capital has emerged in the literature as a valuable concept to understanding inequality, including health disparities [32-34]. It has been used to examine the unequal distribution of social resources available to individuals within their communities and across social networks [35-37]. In recent years, social capital has been joined with the concept of "community" in an effort to promote "community as the site where responsibility for ameliorating social problems lies" [38].

In this paper, we define social capital as the resources of individuals in social relationships as well as the resources within their social networks and community [39]. Two key dimensions of social capital are perceived social cohesion and perceived social disorder. Social capital, specifically perceived social cohesion, has been associated negatively with gonorrhea rates [40,41] and increased odds of condom use at last sex among African American youth [42]. However, a qualitative investigation that highlighted the presence of positive role models as a form of social capital found that the lack of such role models was perceived to increase HIV risk-taking [43]. Similarly, a study on gang membership also found it to reduce HIV protective behaviors [41]. Whereas gang membership likely results in social capital, especially perceived social cohesion, it also may encourage behaviors that place a person at risk for HIV (e.g., social norms unsupportive of condom use result in unsafe sex). Yet others found that women who ceased using drugs and no longer engaged in transactional sex to pay for their habit increasingly became alienated from their social and sexual networks [44]. Hence, as their HIV risk-taking decreased, their social capital did so as well.

Perceived social disorder, our second dimension of social capital, has also been associated with sexual risk-taking. For example, findings from recent studies show a link between social disorder (e.g., public drinking and visible drug sales and use) and increased rates of sexually transmitted infections (STIs) [41, 45]. Additionally, perceptions of violence and homicide rates have also been associated with increased STI rates [41].

Substance use and condom use

Substance use as a risk factor for unprotected sex arises in the context of relationships and sexual partnerships, as a correlate of socioeconomic status and as a characteristic of the social environment, making it an important situational construct to consider. The use of alcohol and other drugs has been associated with unprotected sex [46,47]. However, interesting gender differences emerge and it seems that the interaction of alcohol use by partner type and unsafe sex holds for women but to a more limited extent for men as men may have more direct control over condom use than women [48]. For example, binge drinking has been associated with increased STI incidence among women seeking treatment at a clinic although the association was not found for men [46].

Similar dynamics may come into play when drugs other than alcohol are being used. Female drug users tend to be more stigmatized by their male counterparts as well as by society-at-large [7]. Others have challenged the link between the use of alcohol and other drugs and the lack of condom use, especially when exploring this at the event level [18]. Among users of illicit drugs, recent findings show unsafe sex to be related to the use of certain types of drugs (e.g., cocaine, methamphetamine and amphetamine) but not other drugs (e.g., marijuana and heroin) among drug-offending males [47].

Finally, researchers found that the setting in which drugs are being used and in which sex occurs influences condom use [49]. For example, use in a crack house in which the norms allow for the exchange of sex for crack tends not to involve condom use. This may account for why recent crack use has demonstrated an association with reduced odds of condom use among low-income women [17].

The multi-domain approach of this study, including proximate and more distal factors, guides our inquiry to assess independent correlates of the lack of condom use during vaginal sex with primary partners, while controlling for substance use. We consider relationships and sexual partnerships as a key proximal domain and socio-economic status and social capital as more distal domains. By adding to the current knowledge about the dynamics regarding the lack of condom use with primary partners, we hope to contribute to ongoing efforts to reduce the health disparities, specifically those related to HIV/AIDS, faced by poor African Americans who reside in inner-city neighborhoods with limited social capital.

Our study

Data for this chapter were collected as part of People and Places, a cross-sectional study of people and their perceptions of how their neighborhood impacted their daily lives and actions. Data were collected between May 2009 and August 2011 in Atlanta, Georgia. Participants (n=1,050) were recruited from 77 census block groups, using active community outreach strategies (e.g., recruiting directly in neighborhoods or via key respondents) and passive methods, specifically by posting flyers. The sampling frame was designed to ensure sufficient variability by gender, age, and drug use.

Eligible respondents self-identified as African American, were at least age 18, and had lived in the same neighborhood for the past year. Additional eligibility criteria for this paper were having had vaginal sex with a primary partner in the past 30 days and self-reporting as HIV-negative. The sexual activity criterion was added to ensure that we would be able to explore condom use behaviors in the context of vaginal sex in the past 30 days. A negative HIV status was included as a means of recognizing that condom use among HIV negative individuals serves as a main means to protect against HIV acquisition.

The survey included demographics, psychosocial characteristics, licit and illicit drug use history, sexual activity history, criminal justice involvement, and neighborhood perceptions. The Emory University Institutional Review Board approved the study protocol. Interviews lasted approximately 90 minutes and were conducted in a private office at the study site, which was located in one of the neighborhoods. Participants were compensated $30 for their time.

Measures

Outcome measure: Lack of Condom Use during Vaginal Sex with Primary Partners was derived from two questions. Participants were asked the number of times they engaged in any type of sex with primary partners in the past 30 days prior to the interview and then the question: "Of the [insert number of times] that you had vaginal sex with a primary partner or partners in the past 30 days, how many times did you or your partner use a male condom?" The responses were dichotomized as no condom use (1) and having used condoms at least once (0).

Demographics: Gender was self-identified as "male" (0) and "female" (1). Age (in years) was calculated using the participant's date of birth and the date of the interview.

Use of alcohol and other drugs: Alcohol use, crack/cocaine use and marijuana use in the past 30 days were dichotomized with 0=No and 1=Yes. Crack/cocaine and marijuana were selected in addition to alcohol due their prevalence in the Atlanta area [50].

Relationship and sexual partnership: Partnered was coded as not having a partner (0) or being with a partner, regardless of the living situation (1). The importance of a relationship with a primary partner was dichotomized into it being important (1) versus it not being important (0). Participants were asked about number of sexual partners by type of partner (primary, casual, and paid or paying) during the last 30 days. For this study, multiple partners was conceptualized as a three-level variable: having one primary partner, having more than one primary partner and possibly other types of partners, or only one primary partner with other types of partners. Given the focus on condom use with primary partners, which is least likely to be the case as compared with other partner types, each response option includes primary partners.

Socioeconomic status: Income was measured through a series of questions about the amount of income received in the past 30 days from a variety of sources including legal employment, "under the table" income, public assistance, retirement benefits, unemployment benefits, family sources, illegal income, and other sources. A total was calculated and the participant was asked to confirm the amount. For the purposes of this study, the square root of income was computed to make the variable conform to a normal distribution. The square root was applied as it resulted in a less skewed and less kurtotic transformed variable then taking the natural log. Employed reflected the respondent's current employment status and was dichotomized as not being employed (0) and being employed, either full or part-time (1). Homelessness was dichotomized as never having been homeless (0) to ever having been homeless (1). Educational attainment was captured by dichotomizing the responses between less than a high school education (0) and a high school education (including GED) or greater (1). Having health insurance was measured as no or inconsistent health insurance coverage in the past 12 months (0) versus having had health insurance coverage for all of the last 12 months (1). Current living situation was assessed as residing in your own house, condominium, townhome, or apartment (1) versus not having your own residence (0).

Social capital: Perceived social cohesion was measured using a 5-item scale [51] with questions such as "How often do you and people in your neighborhood do favors for each other?" and "How often do you and other people in the neighborhood ask each other for advice about personal things, such as child-rearing or job-openings?" (Cronbach's alpha = .78). Item responses ranged from 0=Never to 3=Often and scores were summed such that higher scores corresponded to greater perception of social cohesion. Perceived neighborhood disorder was assessed with a 7-item scale [52] that included statements such as "In my neighborhood, people watch out for each other" and "Police protection in my neighborhood is adequate" (alpha=.81). One item from the original scale was removed due to its similarity to perceived social cohesion. Response options ranged from 0=Strongly Disagree to 4=Strongly Agree. Higher scores corresponded to greater perceived disorder. Knowledge of crime in the neighborhood was measured by asking if the respondent knew if any of a series of violent events (e.g., shooting, sexual assault, robbery, or mugging) occurred in their neighborhood during the past 6 months, with responses ranged from never (0) to often (3) (alpha=. 71). Observed violence in the neighborhood was measured with seven questions from the Community Experiences Questionnaire [53]. The items addressed having observed in the neighborhood during the past year events such as "somebody got hit, punched, or slapped" and "somebody got arrested or taken away by the police". Response options ranged from never (0) to often (3). Higher scores corresponded to greater levels of having observed violence (alpha=. 87).

Analysis

Generalized estimating equations (GEE) applying a logit link were used to conduct logistic regression with the software package SPSS Statistics 19. The respondents were sampled by a census block group and GEE were used because they provide a means of accounting for the correlation between people within these groups. GEE calculates the standard errors of parameter estimates based upon the within-cluster similarity of the residuals [54] thereby providing more accurate confidence intervals. Crude odds ratios were calculated and variables found to be significant at the level of $p < .10$ were included in the multivariate analysis. Missing data were minimal (2.6%) and any cases lacking a variable included in the multivariate model were dropped for that analysis. A sensitivity analysis was also conducted with respect to the outcome variable of a lack of condom use. It has been asserted that grouping the "sometimes users" of condoms with the "always" users of condoms or "never" users of condoms can lead to inaccurate assessment of statistical associations [55]. To avoid such errors, the alternate proportion of always using condoms versus sometimes or never using condoms was tested as the outcome in multivariate analysis and the analysis revealed that the results did not alter the basic conclusions of the study.

Our findings

Descriptive statistics are displayed in table 1. The study sample included nearly equal proportions of men and women (49% and 51%) and 51% were over the age of 35. The age of 35 is used as a cut-off because we are interested in exploring the impact of drug use. Drug researchers tend to refer to those over 35 as older [56].

Being over 35 was associated with increases in the odds of the lack of condom use when engaging in vaginal sex in the past 30 days with primary partners (hereafter referred to as "lack of condom use"). Alcohol use demonstrated a trend toward a positive association with a lack of condom use, whereas crack cocaine or marijuana use was not associated with lack of condom use. The relationship and sexual partnership characteristics demonstrated significant associations with the lack of condom use: having a partner and considering a primary relationship to be important were associated positively with a lack of condom use, while having more than one primary partner (but not having other types of partners in addition to a single primary partner) was associated negatively with a lack of condom use compared to having only one primary partner. In the domain of socioeconomic status, having ever been homeless was associated with an increase in the odds of a lack of condom use, while having health insurance was associated with a decrease in the odds of a lack of condom use. Among the social capital indicators, perceived social cohesion was associated with a decrease in the odds of a lack of condom use, but perceived neighborhood disorder was associated with an increase in the odds of a lack of condom use.

Table 1. Descriptive statistics and crude odds ratios (n=1050)

Variable	Mean (SD)/ Number (%)	Lack of Condoms Past 30 Days with Primary Partners	
		OR	95% CI
Never Use of Condoms Primary Partners	.57		
Demographics			
Gender	.51	1.09	(0.88, 1.35)
Age (>35)	.51	2.12	(1.70, 2.65)***
Use of Alcohol and Other Drugs			
Alcohol Past 30 Days	.71	1.27	(0.96, 1.68)†
Crack/Cocaine Past 30 Days	.27	1.17	(0.91, 1.52)
Marijuana Past 30 Days	.52	0.96	(0.75, 1.23)
Relationship and Sexual Partnerships			
Partnered	.74	2.82	(2.12, 3.74)***
Primary Partner Important	.78	1.86	(1.39, 2.48)***
Multiple Partners[a]			
At least two primary partners	.10	0.20	(0.12, 0.34)***
Only one primary partner with other partners	.10	0.99	(0.62, 1.56)
Socioeconomic Status			
Income[b]	25.75 (13.72)	1.00	(0.99, 1.01)
Employed	.23	0.89	(0.67, 1.18)
Homeless	.37	1.63	(1.27, 2.08)***
High school	.60	1.09	(0.83, 1.44)
Health Insurance[c]	.36	0.73	(0.56, 0.95)*
Own Home	.10	0.93	(0.61, 1.41)
Social Capital			
Perceived Social Cohesion	9.08 (3.91)	0.96	(0.93, 0.99)*
Perceived Neighborhood Disorder	16.11 (5.57)	1.03	(1.00, 1.05)*
Knowledge of Crime	3.79 (2.53)	1.00	(0.95, 1.06)
Observed Crime	11.37 (5.88)	1.00	(0.98, 1.02)

† $p < .10$, * $p < .05$, ** $p < .01$, *** $p < .001$.
[a] Reference category is having only one primary partner.
[b] Square root transformed.
[c] Reference category is not having health insurance consistently over the past 12 months.

Table 2 includes the variables that were associated significantly with a lack of condom use at the level of $p < .10$ in bivariate analysis. In multivariate analysis, being older than 35 was associated with an increase in the odds of a lack of condom use. The relationship variables were associated significantly with the outcome variable also. Both being partnered (OR=2.64; CI: 1.96, 3.54) and considering having a primary partner to be important (OR=1.35; CI: 1.02, 1.81) were associated positively with a lack of condom use. Having more than one primary partner and possibly other types of partners compared to having only one primary partner in the past 30 days was protective against a lack of condom use (OR=0.22; CI: 0.13, 0.36). However, having only one primary partner and other types of partners compared to having only one primary partner was not associated with a lack of condom use.

Table 2. Adjusted odds ratios

	Lack of Condoms Past 30 Days with Primary Partners (n=1023)	
Variable	OR	95% CI[a]
Demographics		
Age (>35)	2.12	(1.61, 2.79)***
Use of Alcohol and Other Drugs		
Alcohol Past 30 Days	1.12	(0.80, 1.55)
Relationship and Sexual Partnerships		
Partnered	2.64	(1.96, 3.54)***
Primary Partner Important	1.35	(1.02, 1.81)*
Multiple Partners[a]		
At least two primary partners	0.22	(0.13, 0.36)***
Only one primary partner with other partners	1.08	(0.66, 1.78)
Socioeconomic Status		
Homeless	1.38	(1.06, 1.81)*
Health Insurance[b]	0.71	(0.52, 0.96)*
Social Capital		
Perceived Social Cohesion	0.96	(0.92, 0.99)*
Perceived Neighborhood Disorder	1.02	(1.00, 1.05)†

† p < .10, * p < .05, ** p < .01, *** p < .001.

[a] Reference category is having only one primary partner.

[b] Reference category is not having health insurance consistently over the past 12 months.

The domains of socioeconomic status and social capital also revealed significant associations with a lack of condom use. Ever having been homeless was associated positively (OR: 1.38, CI: 1.06, 1.81) with the outcome variable, while having health insurance consistently over the past 12 months was associated negatively (OR: 0.71, CI: 0.52, 0.96) with the outcome variable. An increase in perceived social cohesion was associated with reduced odds of lack of condom use with a primary partner (OR: 0.96; CI: 0.92, 0.99).

Discussion

In this study, we examine the impact of relationship and sexual partnership factors as well as more distal social factors on a lack of condom use when engaging in vaginal sex with primary partners among African American men and women. A majority of the sample (57%) reported not having used a condom when having vaginal sex with a primary partner in the past 30 days prior to the interview. A lack of condom use with primary partners is commonly reported in the literature [29,57], due to a partner's negative attitude toward condoms [57] and the association of condom use with a lack of trust and love [21]. Our findings show that being partnered and perceiving to have a primary partner as important were associated positively with a lack of condom use, the latter independent of relationship status. Considering having a primary partner as important may result in unsafe behaviors, without considering the potential HIV status of the partner or recognizing that many individuals are unaware of their HIV status [58]. A second concern is that the decision not to use condoms may be based on the assumption that a primary partner is not having sex with other people [59]. In the literature, concurrent sexual partnerships have been highlighted as contributing to the HIV epidemic, especially among African American men and women [60].

It has been asserted that examining not only the individual but also the nature of the partnership is necessary to improve the understanding of HIV acquisition, particularly as it relates to concurrent partnerships [57]. In this study, one-fifth of the participants reported having more than one partner in the past 30 days. Among those who reported more than one primary partner (compared to having only one primary partner) in the past 30 days a negative association was found in the odds of a lack of condom use with primary partners. However, for study participants who indicated having had at least one primary and additional non-primary partner (e.g., casual or transactional partners) compared to having only one primary partner, no association was found with the lack of condom use with primary partners. Past qualitative research findings also showed the importance of differentiating between the patterns of concurrent relationships [61]. That study showed that people in multiple partnerships used condoms only with partners other than their "primary" or primary partners in most situations. The failure to show an association between having only one primary partner in addition to other types of partners and a lack of condom use with primary partners is consistent with those findings. Condom use within the primary partnership would not be impacted by additional partners. However, the results of the current study also imply that if more than one person is considered primary that demarcation may not preclude condom use with primary partners.

Beyond the relationship and sexual partnerships, we found condom use to be impacted by dimensions from more distal domains. The socioeconomic factor of ever having been homeless was associated positively with a lack of condom use. Experiencing homelessness may represent acute economic deprivation and reduce concerns about future HIV acquisition due to a lack of condom use [17]. Having health insurance during the past 12 months also was associated negatively with a lack of condom use. It may be that those who have health insurance are more likely to seek regular health checks and exhibit healthy behaviors more generally. For example, a study of a national sample of women found that women who had health insurance were more likely to have received health checks such as a pap smear [62].

The domain of social capital revealed an association between perceived social cohesion and a reduction in the odds of a lack of condom use. This finding is consistent with previous research that has found that social cohesion exhibited a protective effect against HIV risk behaviors [40,42]. Other dimensions of social capital were not associated with a lack of condom use, possibly because these are too distal for our inquiry.

Substance use was not associated with a lack of condom use. This is not unexpected given that drinking in particular is more often associated with condom use with non-primary partners [18,63]. It may also be that situational factors do not impact condom use with primary partners because condom use is not prevalent with primary or regular partners in general [29,57].

Limitations

This study has a number of limitations. The sampling approach is not a random sampling strategy and there may be an inherent bias in who was enrolled in People and Places [64]. All interviews were conducted in the Atlanta, Georgia metropolitan area. There may very well be local or regional influences or subcultural differences between these participants and those residing elsewhere that could affect the generalizability of the data.

Sexual behavior represents a sensitive topic that may be subject to respondent social desirability bias. Given the fact that sexual behavior was assessed based on self-report, the extent to which respondents under or over-reported their behaviors is unknown. Nevertheless, others have shown information on (e.g., sexual behaviors, alcohol consumption, and drug use) to be valid [65-68]. Another potential limitation of the self-reported information is recall bias. We focused mainly on the time frame of the "past 30 days" as a means to minimize recall bias. Although we are unable to determine the extent to which recall bias affected the data, others who conducted research on similar topics reported that bias is sufficiently nominal that its impact upon study findings is likely to be minimal [69].

The cross-sectional design precludes any causal inferences. Among the measures, the non-primary partners included both casual and paid or paying partners; and these two alternatives to primary partners may be qualitatively different. Overall, there is a need for more refined research on partner types. The analysis also did not account for same sex partnerships, as the focus was heterosexual vaginal sex given the salience of this behavior for the HIV/AIDS rates among African Americans. Finally, we only examined the concurrency status of the participants. It would be useful to include a measure of their perception of whether their partners also have additional partners to better understand the nature of the relationship and how it relates to a lack of condom use with primary partners.

Social science implications

Given that a lack of condom use when engaging in vaginal sex with primary partners during the past 30 days is prevalent, factors beyond the individual and outside the interpersonal domain become more important. Much attention has been paid to the economic disparities among African Americans in the United States; this study accounts for the importance of socioeconomic status when assessing the lack of condom use in this specific type of partnership. Patterns of deprivation have been linked to concurrency among African Americans [60] and increase the importance of identifying specific aspects of disparities that are associated with a lack of condom use with primary partners. The results of this study suggest that it is not only extreme indicators such as the experience of homelessness, but also access to health resources such as health insurance, that influence whether one will consider using condoms with a primary partner. These findings also indicate that not only personal but also collective resources, such as perceived social cohesion, impact a lack of condom use with primary partners. Trust and reciprocity within social networks have been associated with health and psychological well-being more generally [70], and may contribute to health-related decision-making involving condom use. Factors outside the partnership (e.g., social and sexual network norms) provide potential pathways to increasing the use of condoms even in primary partnerships where a lack of condom use is the norm [13,29].

The multi-domain approach to understanding why people do or do not use condoms with certain partners is typical of sociological inquiry. In addressing our research question, we aimed to provide an epistemology of the HIV-related health disparities experienced by African Americans. We show how factors beyond the individual impact actions, in this case, the influence of socioeconomic characteristics and social capital. These tap into the position of the individual in society (e.g., homelessness and having health insurance) as well as the conditions of the neighborhood in which one resides. Recently, public health has gained an appreciation for the importance of social capital, specifically social cohesion and our findings support this path of inquiry. It is through this type of epistemology that social science may make contributions; it shows the importance of considering epidemiological information in the larger socio-political and ecological context.

Acknowledgments

This research was supported by funding from the National Institute on Drug Abuse RO1DA025607 and RO1DA25949) and the Center for AIDS Research at Emory University (P30AI050409). The views presented are those of the authors.

References

[1] CDC. *Acquired immunodeficiency syndrome (AIDS) among blacks and Hispanics--United States. MMWR*, 1986;35(42):655-8,663-6.

[2] CDC. *HIV among African Americans.* 2010. Retrieved from http://www.cdc.gov/hiv/topics/aa/pdf/aa.pdf.

[3] CDC. Estimated lifetime risk for diagnosis of HIV infection among Hispanics/Latinos--37 states and Puerto Rico, 2007. *MMWR* 2010;59(40):1297-301.

[4] Marshall P, Singer M, Clatts M. Integrating cultural, observational, and epidemiological approaches in the prevention of drug abuse and HIV/AIDS. *NIDA Monograph.* Washington, DC: Government Printing Office, 1999:97-115.

[5] Singer M. AIDS and the health crisis of the US urban poor: The perspective of critical medical anthropology. *Soc. Sci. Med.* 1994;39:931-48.

[6] Singer M. *Introduction to syndemics: A systems approach to public and community health.* San Francisco, CA: Jossey-Bass, 2009.

[7] Sterk C. *Fast lives: Women who use crack cocaine.* Philadelphia, PA: Temple University Press, 1999.

[8] Aral SO, Adimora AA, Fenton KA. Understanding and responding to disparities in HIV and other sexually transmitted infections in African Americans. *Lancet,* 2008;372(9635):337-40.

[9] CDC. *Estimates of new HIV infections in the United States,* 2006-2009. 2011. Retrieved from http://www.cdc.gov/hiv/topics/surveillance/factsheets.htm.

[10] Harrison KM, Dean HD. Use of data systems to address social determinants of health: A need to do more. *Public Health Rep.,* 2011;126(Suppl 3):1-5.

[11] White House Office of National AIDS Policy. *National HIV/AIDS strategy*. 2010. Retrieved from http://aids.gov/federal-resources/policies/national-hiv-aids-strategy/nhas.pdf.

[12] Dancy BL, Berbaum ML. Condom use predictors for low-income African American women. *West J. Nurs. Res.* 2005;27(1):28-44.

[13] Macaluso M, Demand MJ, Artz LM, Hook EWI. Partner type and condom use. *AIDS* 2000;14(5):537-46.

[14] Catania J, Coates TJ, Kegeles S. A test of the AIDS Risk Reduction Model: Psychosocial correlates of condom use in the AMEN cohort survey. *Health Psychol.* 1994;13(6):548-55.

[15] Wingood G, DiClemente R. Partner influences and gender-related factors associated with non-condom use among young adult African American women. *Am. J. Community Psychol* 1998;26:29-51.

[16] Lichtenstein B, Desmond RA, Schwebke JR. Partnership concurrency status and condom use among women diagnosed with trichomonas vaginalis. *Womens Health Issues* 2008;18(5):369-74.

[17] Ober A, Iguchi M, Weiss R, Gorbach P, Heimer R, Ouellet L, et al. The relative role of perceived partner risks in promoting condom use in a three-city sample of high-risk, low-income women. *AIDS Behav.* 2011;15(7):1347-58.

[18] Scott-Sheldon L, Carey M, Vanable P, Senn T, Coury-Doniger P, Urban M. Alcohol consumption, drug use, and condom use among STD clinic patients. *J. Stud. Alcohol* 2009;70(5):762-70.

[19] Schilling R, El-Bassel N, Schinke S, Gordon K, Nichols S. Building skills of recovering women drug users to reduce heterosexual AIDS transmission. *Public Health Rep.* 1991;106:297-304.

[20] Theall KP, Sterk CE, Elifson KW. Male condom use by type of relationships following an HIV intervention among women who use illegal drugs. *J. Drug Issues* 2003;33:1-28.

[21] Corbett AM, Dickson-Gómez J, Hilario H, Weeks MR. A little thing called love: Condom use in high-risk primary heterosexual relationships. Perspect *Sex Reprod. Health* 2009;41(4):218-24.

[22] Allen M, Emmers-Sommer TM, Crowell TL. Couples negotiating safer sex behaviors: A meta-analysis of the impact of conversation and gender. In: Allen M, Preiss RW, Gayle BM, Burrell NA, editors. *Interpersonal communication research: Advances through meta-analysis*. Mahwah, NJ: Lawrence Erlbaum, 2002:263-79.

[23] Noar SM, Morokoff PJ, Harlow LL. Condom negotiation in heterosexually active men and women: Development and validation of a condom influence strategy questionnaire. *Psychol. Health* 2002;17:711-35.

[24] Aida Y, Falbo T. Relationships between marital satisfaction, resources, and power strategies. *Sex Roles* 1991;24(1/2):43-56.

[25] Noar SM, Zimmerman RS, Atwood KA. Safer sex and sexually transmitted infections from a relationship perspective. In: Harvey JH, Wenzel A, Sprecher S, editors. *Handbook of sexuality in close relationships*. Mahwah, NJ: Lawrence Erlbaum, 2004:519-44.

[26] Ickovics J, Yoshikawa H. Preventive interventions to reduce heterosexual HIV risk for women: Current perspectives, future directions. *AIDS* 1998;12:S197-208.

[27] Adimora AA, Schoenbach VJ. Social context, sexual networks, and racial disparities in rates of sexually transmitted infections. *J. Infect. Dis.* 2005;191(Suppl 1):S115-S22.

[28] Magnus M, Kuo I, Shelley K, Rawls A, Peterson J, Montanez L, et al. Risk factors driving the emergence of a generalized heterosexual HIV epidemic in Washington, District of Columbia networks at risk. *AIDS* 2009;23(10):1277-84.

[29] Senn TE, Carey MP, Vanable PA, Coury-Doniger P, Urban M. Sexual partner concurrency among STI clinic patients with a steady partner: Correlates and associations with condom use. *Sex Transm. Dis.* 2009;85(5):343-7.

[30] Ford JL, Browning CR. Neighborhood social disorganization and the acquisition of trichomoniasis among young adults in the United States. *Am. J. Public Health* 2011;101(9):1696-703.

[31] Dunkle K, Wingood G, Camp C, DiClemente R. Economically motivated relationships and transactional sex among unmarried African American and white women: Results from a U.S. national telephone survey. *Public Health Rep.* 2010;125(S4):90-125.

[32] Schuller T. Reflections of the use of social capital. *Rev. Soc. Econ.* 2007;65(1):11-28.

[33] Lockhart WH. Building bridges and bonds: Generating social capital in secular and faith based poverty-to-work programs. *Sociol. Relig.* 2005;66(1):45-60.

[34] Putnam RD. *Bowling alone: The collapse and revival of american community.* New York, NY: Simon Schuster, 2000.

[35] Bourdieu P. *Distinction: A social critique of the judgement of taste.* Cambridge, MA: Harvard University Press, 1984.

[36] Coleman JS. Social capital in the creation of human capital. *Am. J. Sociol.* 1988;94:95-121.

[37] Lin N. *Social capital: A theory of social structure and action.* Cambridge, MA: University Press, 2001.

[38] Bryson L, Mowbray M. More spray on solution: Community, social capital and evidence based policy. *Aust. J. Soc. Issues* 2005;40(1):91-106.

[39] Thomas-Slayter BP, Fisher WF. Social capital and AIDS-resilient communities: Strengthening the AIDS response. Glob Public Health 2011:1-21.

[40] Ellen JM, Jennings JM, Meyers T, Chung S-E, Taylor R. Perceived social cohesion and prevalence of sexually transmitted diseases. *Sex Transm. Dis.* 2004;31(2):117-22.

[41] Thomas J, Torrone E, Browning C. Neighborhood factors affecting rates of sexually transmitted diseases in Chicago. *J. Urban Health* 2010;87(1):102-12.

[42] Kerrigan D, Witt S, Glass B, Chung S-e, Ellen J. Perceived neighborhood social cohesion and condom use among adolescents vulnerable to HIV/STI. *AIDS Behav.* 2006;10(6):723-9.

[43] Cené C, Akers A, Lloyd S, Albritton T, Powell Hammond W, Corbie-Smith G. Understanding social capital and HIV risk in rural African American communities. *J. Gen. Intern Med.* 2011;26(7):737-44.

[44] Sterk C, Elifson K, Theall K. Individual action and community context: The health intervention project. *Am. J. Prev. Med.* 2007;32(Suppl 6):S177-S81.

[45] Lang D, Salazar L, Crosby R, DiClemente R, Brown L, Donenberg G. Neighborhood environment, sexual risk behaviors and acquisition of sexually transmitted infections among adolescents diagnosed with psychological disorders. *Am. J. Community Psychol.* 2010;46(3):303-11.

[46] Hutton HE, McCaul ME, Santora PB, Erbelding EJ. The relationship between recent alcohol use and sexual behaviors: Gender differences among sexually transmitted disease clinic patients. *Alcohol Clin. Exp. Res.* 2008;32(11):2008-15.

[47] Leigh B, Stall R. Substance use and risky sexual behavior for exposure to HIV: Issues in methodology, interpretation, and prevention. *Am. Psychol.* 1993;48:1035-45.

[48] Pulerwitz J, Amaro H, Jong WD, Gortmaker SL, Rudd R. Relationship power, condom use and HIV risk among women in the USA. *AIDS Care* 2002;14(6):789-800.

[49] Kopetz CE, Reynolds EK, Hart CL, Kruglanski AW, Lejuez CW. Social context and perceived effects of drugs on sexual behavior among individuals who use both heroin and cocaine. *Exp. Clin. Psychopharmacol.* 2010;18(3):214-20.

[50] DePadilla L, Wolfe M. Drug abuse patterns and trends in Atlanta--Update: June 2010. *Epidemiologic Trends in Drug Abuse: Proceedings of the Community Epidemiology Work Group.* Bethesda, MD: US Department Health Human Services, 2010.

[51] Sampson RJ, Morenoff JD, Felton E. Beyond social capital: Spatial dynamics of collective efficacy for children. *Am. Sociol. Rev.* 1999;64(5):633-60.

[52] Ross CE, Mirowsky J. *Disorder and decay. Urban Aff. Rev.,* 1999;34(3):412-32.

[53] Schwartz D, Proctor LJ. Community violence exposure and children's social adjustment in the school peer group: The mediating roles of emotion regulation and social cognition. *J. Consult Clin. Psychol.* 2000;68(4):670-83.

[54] Hanley JA, Negassa A, Edwardes MDd, Forrester JE. Statistical analysis of correlated data using generalized estimating equations: An orientation. *Am. J. Epidemiol.* 2003;157(4):364-75.

[55] Crosby R, DiClemente RJ, Holtgrave DR, Wingood GM. Design, measurement, and analytical considerations for testing hypotheses relative to condom effectiveness against non-viral STIs. *Sex Transm. Infect.* 2002;78(4):228-31.

[56] Gfroerer J, Penne M, Pembertin M, Folsom R. Substance abuse treatment need among older adults in 2020: The impact of the aging baby-boom cohort. *Drug Alcohol Depend* 2003;69:127-35.

[57] Gorbach P, Holmes KK. Transmission of STIs/HIV at the partnership level: Beyond individual-level analyses. *J. Urban Health* 2003; 80(0):iii15-iii25.

[58] Campsmith ML, Rhodes PH, Hall I, Green TA. Undiagnosed HIV prevalence among adults and adolescents in the United States at the end of 2006. *J. Acquir Immune Defic. Syndr.* 2010;53(5):619-24.

[59] Drumright LN, Gorbach PM, Holmes KK. Do people really know their sex partners?: Concurrency, knowledge of partner behavior, and sexually transmitted infections within partnerships. *Sex Transm. Dis.* 2004;31(7):437-42.

[60] Adimora AA, Schoenbach VJ, Doherty IA. HIV and African Americans in the southern United States: Sexual networks and social context. *Sex Transm. Dis.* 2006;33(7):S39-S45.

[61] Gorbach P, Stoner BP, Aral SO, H. Whittington WL, Holmes K. "It takes a village": Understanding concurrent sexual partnerships in Seattle, Washington. *Sex Transm. Dis.* 2002;29(8):453-62.

[62] Coughlin SS, Leadbetter S, Richards T, Sabatino SA. Contextual analysis of breast and cervical cancer screening and factors associated with health care access among United States women, 2002. *Soc. Sci. Med.* 2008;66(2):260-75.

[63] Raj A, Reed E, Santana MC, Walley AY, Welles SL, Horsburgh CR, et al. The associations of binge alcohol use with HIV/STI risk and diagnosis among heterosexual African American men. *Drug Alcohol Depend* 2009;101(1-2):101-6.

[64] Heckathorn DD. Respondent-Driven Sampling: A New Approach to the Study of Hidden Populations. *Soc. Problems* 1997;44(2):174-99.

[65] Anglin M, Hser Y, Chou C. Reliability and validity of retrospective behavioral self-report by narcotics addicts. *Evaluation Rev.* 1993;17:91-103.

[66] Higgins ST, Budney AJ, Bickel WK, Badger GJ, Foerg FE, Ogden D. Outpatient behavioral treatment for cocaine dependence: One-year outcome. *Exp. Clin. Psychopharmacol.* 1995;3(2):205-12.

[67] Miller M, Paone D. Social network characteristics as mediators in the relationship between sexual abuse and HIV risk. *Soc. Sci. Med.* 1998;47(6):765-77.

[68] Nurco DN. *A discussion of validity: Self-report methods of estimating drug use.* Washinfgton, DC: NIDA Res Monogr 57, US Government Printing Office, 1985:4-11.

[69] Jaccard J, Wan CK. A paradigm for studying the accuracy of self-reports of risk behavior relevant to AIDS: Empirical perspectives on stability, recall bias, and transitory influences. *J. Appl. Soc. Psychol.* 1995;25:1831-58.

[70] Nieminen T, Martelin T, Koskinen S, Aro H, Alanen E, Hyyppä M. Social capital as a determinant of self-rated health and psychological well-being. *Int. J. Public Health,* 2010;55(6):531-42.

Acknowledgments

ISBN 978-1-62081-293-8

Chapter VIII

About the editors

Hugh Klein, PhD has a joint affiliation with Kensington Research Institute, Silver Spring, Maryland and Emory University in Atlanta, Georgia, where he works as a senior researcher in the Rollins School of Public Health. He is a sociologist who earned his PhD from Washington University in St. Louis in 1990. His main research interests and areas of expertise are in the fields of substance use/abuse, HIV/AIDS, the mass media, sexual health, the use of new media technologies to promote health, and prevention/intervention research. He is the author of one book, several book chapters, and more than 60 publications in peer-reviewed journals, and has been an author of more than 150 papers at various regional, national, and international conferences, such as the American Sociological Association, American Public Health Association, College on Problems of Drug Dependence, and Society for the Study of Social Problems. E-mail: hughk@aol.com (primary) or hughkhughk@yahoo.com (secondary).

Joav Merrick, MD, MMedSci, DMSc, is professor of pediatrics, child health and human development affiliated with Kentucky Children's Hospital, University of Kentucky, Lexington, United States and the Division of Pediatrics, Hadassah Hebrew University Medical Centers, Mt Scopus Campus, Jerusalem, Israel, the medical director of the Health Services, Division for Intellectual and Developmental Disabilities, Ministry of Social Affairs and Social Services, Jerusalem, the founder and director of the National Institute of Child Health and Human Development in Israel. Numerous publications in the field of pediatrics, child health and human development, rehabilitation, intellectual disability, disability, health, welfare, abuse, advocacy, quality of life and prevention. Received the Peter Sabroe Child Award for outstanding work on behalf of Danish Children in 1985 and the International LEGO-Prize ("The Children's Nobel Prize") for an extraordinary contribution towards improvement in child welfare and wellbeing in 1987. E-mail: jmerrick@zahav.net.il

In: Human Immunodeficiency Virus …
Editor: Hugh Klein and Joav Merrick
ISBN 978-1-62081-293-8

Chapter IX

About the Kensington Research Institute, Silver Spring, Maryland, United States

Kensington Research Institute (KRI) was established in 1993. The company is devoted to conducting social science research, health services research, intervention research, prevention studies and providing a broad array of support services for evaluation researchers. Corporate specializations encompass the fields of HIV/AIDS, substance use and abuse, women's health, children's and adolescent health, family violence (e.g., sexual abuse, physical abuse, emotional abuse, neglect), and the media.

Research activities

Since its establishment in the mid-1990s, KRI, primarily through the work of Dr. Hugh Klein, has been involved in a wide variety of research projects that have examined the nexus of substance use/abuse, mental health functioning, and HIV/AIDS risk practices, as well as a few projects that have focused on mass media influences on social behaviors. Here are a few examples:

- One project, colloquially referred to as *The Cartoons Project*, was a National Institute on Alcohol Abuse and Alcoholism-funded research study of the alcohol-related content of animated cartoons. This project was very broad in scope, examining not only cartoons' messages about alcoholic beverages and drinking, but also an array of other topics that led to publications focusing on cartoons' messages pertaining to 1) body weight, 2) physical attractiveness, 3) race and racism, 4) gender roles, 5) gun violence, 6) physical assault, 7) symbolic annihilation, among others.
- *The Bareback Project* was a National Institute on Drug Abuse-funded initiative designed to study men who use the Internet to find other men for unprotected sex. It utilized a national random sampling strategy to identify, and subsequently recruit, 332 unprotected sex-seeking gay and bisexual men from all over the United States, to find out more about their sexual behaviors, their substance use/abuse practices, and

the myriad factors influencing their risk for HIV. Published articles from this study have focused on such topics as 1) the applicability of syndemics theory to these men's risk practices, 2) substance use and abuse among members of this target population, 3) anonymous sex, 4) differences between younger and older men in terms of their involvement in HIV risk behaviors and the factors underlying their HIV risk, 5) attitudes toward condom use, and 6) childhood maltreatment experiences and their relationship to HIV risk taking in this population.

- *Project FAST (Female Atlanta Study)* was a study undertaken by Drs. Claire Sterk and Kirk Elifson in the Atlanta, Georgia metropolitan area. This research project focused on "at risk" women and examined the interplay of substance use/abuse, psychological and psychosocial functioning, and HIV risk taking. KRI-affiliated published works from this study have focused on 1) self-esteem and HIV risk taking, 2) condom use self-efficacy, 3) temptation to use drugs and actual drug use behaviors, 4) perceived risk for acquiring HIV and its relationship to risk practices, 5) substance abuse problems and HIV risk taking, among others.
- *Project X* was another study undertaken by Drs. Claire Sterk and Kirk Elifson, again in the Atlanta, Georgia metropolitan area. In this study, young adult users of the drug, ecstasy, were interviewed to learn more about the ecstasy experience and the ways that using ecstasy affected young adults' lives. KRI-affiliated works from this study have examined such topics as 1) multiple sex partners, 2) condom use self-efficacy, 3) steps taken to enhance the ecstasy use experience, 4) self-esteem and HIV risk taking and 5) the factors associated with condom use among members of this population.

Collaborations

Since its inception, through its collaborations with other researchers located at other institutions, Kensington Research Institute has been affiliated with several major entities. These include the Department of Sociology at Georgia State University (Atlanta, Georgia), the Rollins School of Public Health at Emory University (Atlanta, Georgia), the Center for Health Disparities Solutions / Prevention Sciences Research Center at Morgan State University (Baltimore, Maryland), the Department of Community and Family Health at University of South Florida (Tampa, Florida), and the Department of Social Welfare at the University of California (Los Angeles, California). KRI-affiliated projects have been funded by the National Institute on Alcohol Abuse and Alcoholism, the National Institute on Drug Abuse, and the National Institute on Minority Health and Health Disparities.

Target populations

As part of its official mission, KRI's research is designed to work with all populations engaging in behaviors that place them at risk for experiencing health and/or social problems. To date, KRI-affiliated projects have targeted an interesting array of "high risk" or "at risk" groups, including:

- children and adolescents
- “at risk” women
- adults aged 18-25 years who use the drug, ecstasy
- adults aged 18-25 years who use powder and/or crack cocaine (as well as members of their immediate family)
- unprotected sex-seeking men who have sex with men
- new users of heroin and/or new users of methamphetamine
- adult persistent smokers
- urban-dwelling African Americans who are “at risk” for drug use/abuse

Contact

Hugh Klein, PhD
Kensington Research institute
401 Schuyler Road
Silver Spring, Maryland 20910 USA
Primary email: hughk@aol.com
Secondary email: hughkhughk@yahoo.com

In: Human Immunodeficiency Virus …
Editor: Hugh Klein and Joav Merrick

ISBN 978-1-62081-293-8

Chapter X

About the National Institute of Child Health and Human Development in Israel

The National Institute of Child Health and Human Development (NICHD) in Israel was established in 1998 as a virtual institute under the auspicies of the Medical Director, Ministry of Social Affairs and Social Services in order to function as the research arm for the Office of the Medical Director. In 1998 the National Council for Child Health and Pediatrics, Ministry of Health and in 1999 the Director General and Deputy Director General of the Ministry of Health endorsed the establishment of the NICHD. In 2011 the NICHD became affiliated with the Division of Pediatrics, Hadassah Hebrew University Medical Centers, Mt Scopus Campus in Jerusalem.

Mission

The mission of a National Institute for Child Health and Human Development in Israel is to provide an academic focal point for the scholarly interdisciplinary study of child life, health, public health, welfare, disability, rehabilitation, intellectual disability and related aspects of human development. This mission includes research, teaching, clinical work, information and public service activities in the field of child health and human development.

Service and academic activities

Over the years many activities became focused in the south of Israel due to collaboration with various professionals at the Faculty of Health Sciences (FOHS) at the Ben Gurion University of the Negev (BGU). Since 2000 an affiliation with the Zusman Child Development Center at the Pediatric Division of Soroka University Medical Center has resulted in collaboration around the establishment of the Down Syndrome Clinic at that center. In 2002 a full course on "Disability" was established at the Recanati School for Allied Professions in the Community, FOHS, BGU and in 2005 collaboration was started with the Primary Care Unit of the faculty and disability became part of the master of public health course on "Children and society". In the academic year 2005-2006 a one-semester course on "Aging with disability" was started as part of the master of science program in gerontology in our collaboration with the Center for Multidisciplinary Research in Aging. In 2010 collaborations with the Division of Pediatrics, Hadassah Medical Centers, Hebrew University, Jerusalem, Israel.

Research activities

The affiliated staff has over the years published work from projects and research activities in this national and international collaboration. In 2000 the International Journal of Adolescent Medicine and Health, and in 2005 the International Journal on Disability and Human development of De Gruyter Publishing House (Berlin and New York), in the year 2003 the TSW-Child Health and Human Development, and in 2006 the TSW-Holistic Health and Medicine of the Scientific World Journal (New York and Kirkkonummi, Finland), all peer-reviewed international journals, were affiliated with the National Institute of Child Health and Human Development. Also, from 2008, the International Journal of Child Health and Human Development (Nova Science, New York), the International Journal of Child and Adolescent Health (Nova Science) and the Journal of Pain Management (Nova Science) were affiliated, and from 2009, the International Public Health Journal (Nova Science) and Journal of Alternative Medicine Research (Nova Science).

National collaborations

Nationally the NICHD works in collaboration with the Faculty of Health Sciences, Ben Gurion University of the Negev; Department of Physical Therapy, Sackler School of Medicine, Tel Aviv University; Autism Center, Assaf HaRofeh Medical Center; National Rett and PKU Centers at Chaim Sheba Medical Center, Tel HaShomer; Department of Physiotherapy, Haifa University; Department of Education, Bar Ilan University, Ramat Gan, Faculty of Social Sciences and Health Sciences; College of Judea and Samaria in Ariel and in 2011 affiliation with Center for Pediatric Chronic Diseases and Center for Down Syndrome, Department of Pediatrics, Hadassah-Hebrew University Medical Center, Mount Scopus Campus, Jerusalem.

International collaborations

Internationally with the Department of Disability and Human Development, College of Applied Health Sciences, University of Illinois at Chicago; Strong Center for Developmental Disabilities, Golisano Children's Hospital at Strong, University of Rochester School of Medicine and Dentistry, New York; Centre on Intellectual Disabilities, University of Albany, New York; Centre for Chronic Disease Prevention and Control, Health Canada, Ottawa;

Chandler Medical Center and Children's Hospital, Kentucky Children's Hospital, Section of Adolescent Medicine, University of Kentucky, Lexington; Chronic Disease Prevention and Control Research Center, Baylor College of Medicine, Houston, Texas; Division of Neuroscience, Department of Psychiatry, Columbia University, New York; Institute for the Study of Disadvantage and Disability, Atlanta; Center for Autism and Related Disorders, Department Psychiatry, Children's Hospital Boston, Boston; Department of Pediatrics, Child Health and Adolescent Medicine, Children's Hospital at Westmead, Westmead, Australia; International Centre for the Study of Occupational and Mental Health, Düsseldorf, Germany; Centre for Advanced Studies in Nursing, Department of General Practice and Primary Care, University of Aberdeen, Aberdeen, United Kingdom; Quality of Life Research Center, Copenhagen, Denmark; Nordic School of Public Health, Gottenburg, Sweden, Scandinavian Institute of Quality of Working Life, Oslo, Norway; Centre for Quality of Life of the Hong Kong Institute of Asia-Pacific Studies and School of Social Work, Chinese University, Hong Kong.

Targets

Our focus is on research, international collaborations, clinical work, teaching and policy in health, disability and human development and to establish the NICHD as a permanent institute at one of the residential care centers for persons with intellectual disability in Israel in order to conduct model research and, together with the four university schools of public health/medicine in Israel, establish a national master and doctoral program in disability and human development at the institute to secure the next generation of professionals working in this often non-prestigious/low-status field of work.

Contact

Joav Merrick, MD, DMSc

Professor of Pediatrics, Child Health and Human Development

Medical Director, Health Services, Division for Intellectual and Developmental Disabilities, Ministry of Social Affairs and Social Services, POB 1260, IL-91012 Jerusalem, Israel.

E-mail: jmerrick@zahav.net.il

In: Human Immunodeficiency Virus …
Editor: Hugh Klein and Joav Merrick
ISBN 978-1-62081-293-8

Chapter XI

About the book series "Health and Human Development"

Health and Human Development is a book series with publications from a multidisciplinary group of researchers, practitioners and clinicians for an international professional forum interested in the broad spectrum of health and human development.

- Merrick J, Omar HA, eds. Adolescent behavior research. International perspectives. New York: Nova Science, 2007.
- Kratky KW. Complementary medicine systems: Comparison and integration. New York: Nova Science, 2008.
- Schofield P, Merrick J, eds. Pain in children and youth. New York: Nova Science, 2009.
- Greydanus DE, Patel DR, Pratt HD, Calles Jr JL, eds. Behavioral pediatrics, 3 ed. New York: Nova Science, 2009.
- Ventegodt S, Merrick J, eds. Meaningful work: Research in quality of working life. New York: Nova Science, 2009.
- Omar HA, Greydanus DE, Patel DR, Merrick J, eds. Obesity and adolescence. A public health concern. New York: Nova Science, 2009.
- Lieberman A, Merrick J, eds. Poverty and children. A public health concern. New York: Nova Science, 2009.
- Goodbread J. Living on the edge. The mythical, spiritual and philosophical roots of social marginality. New York: Nova Science, 2009.
- Bennett DL, Towns S, Elliot E, Merrick J, eds. Challenges in adolescent health: An Australian perspective. New York: Nova Science, 2009.
- Schofield P, Merrick J, eds. Children and pain. New York: Nova Science, 2009.
- Sher L, Kandel I, Merrick J. Alcohol-related cognitive disorders: Research and clinical perspectives. New York: Nova Science, 2009.
- Anyanwu EC. Advances in environmental health effects of toxigenic mold and mycotoxins. New York: Nova Science, 2009.
- Bell E, Merrick J, eds. Rural child health. International aspects. New York: Nova Science, 2009.

- Dubowitz H, Merrick J, eds. International aspects of child abuse and neglect. New York: Nova Science, 2010.
- Shahtahmasebi S, Berridge D. Conceptualizing behavior: A practical guide to data analysis. New York: Nova Science, 2010.
- Wernik U. Chance action and therapy. The playful way of changing. New York: Nova Science, 2010.
- Omar HA, Greydanus DE, Patel DR, Merrick J, eds. Adolescence and chronic illness. A public health concern. New York: Nova Science, 2010.
- Patel DR, Greydanus DE, Omar HA, Merrick J, eds. Adolescence and sports. New York: Nova Science, 2010.
- Shek DTL, Ma HK, Merrick J, eds. Positive youth development: Evaluation and future directions in a Chinese context. New York: Nova Science, 2010.
- Shek DTL, Ma HK, Merrick J, eds. Positive youth development: Implementation of a youth program in a Chinese context. New York: Nova Science, 2010.
- Omar HA, Greydanus DE, Tsitsika AK, Patel DR, Merrick J, eds. Pediatric and adolescent sexuality and gynecology: Principles for the primary care clinician. New York: Nova Science, 2010.
- Chow E, Merrick J, eds. Advanced cancer. Pain and quality of life. New York: Nova Science, 2010.
- Latzer Y, Merrick, J, Stein D, eds. Understanding eating disorders. Integrating culture, psychology and biology. New York: Nova Science, 2010.
- Sahgal A, Chow E, Merrick J, eds. Bone and brain metastases: Advances in research and treatment. New York: Nova Science, 2010.
- Postolache TT, Merrick J, eds. Environment, mood disorders and suicide. New York: Nova Science, 2010.
- Maharajh HD, Merrick J, eds. Social and cultural psychiatry experience from the Caribbean Region. New York: Nova Science, 2010.
- Mirsky J. Narratives and meanings of migration. New York: Nova Science, 2010.
- Harvey PW. Self-management and the health care consumer. New York: Nova Science, 2011.
- Ventegodt S, Merrick J. Sexology from a holistic point of view. New York: Nova Science, 2011.
- Ventegodt S, Merrick J. Principles of holistic psychiatry: A textbook on holistic medicine for mental disorders. New York: Nova Science, 2011.
- Greydanus DE, Calles Jr JL, Patel DR, Nazeer A, Merrick J, eds. Clinical aspects of psychopharmacology in childhood and adolescence. New York: Nova Science, 2011.
- Bell E, Seidel BM, Merrick J, eds. Climate change and rural child health. New York: Nova Science, 2011.
- Bell E, Zimitat C, Merrick J, eds. Rural medical education: Practical strategies. New York: Nova Science, 2011.
- Latzer Y, Tzischinsky. The dance of sleeping and eating among adolescents: Normal and pathological perspectives. New York: Nova Science, 2011.
- Deshmukh VD. The astonishing brain and holistic consciousness: Neuroscience and Vedanta perspectives. New York: Nova Science, 2011.

- Bell E, Westert GP, Merrick J, eds. Translational research for primary healthcare. New York: Nova Science, 2011.
- Shek DTL, Sun RCF, Merrick J, eds. Drug abuse in Hong Kong: Development and evaluation of a prevention program. New York: Nova Science, 2011.
- Ventegodt S, Hermansen TD, Merrick J. Human Development: Biology from a holistic point of view. New York: Nova Science, 2011.
- Ventegodt S, Merrick J. Our search for meaning in life. New York: Nova Science, 2011.
- Caron RM, Merrick J, eds. Building community capacity: Minority and immigrant populations. New York: Nova Science, 2012.

Contact

Professor Joav Merrick, MD, MMedSci, DMSc
Medical Director, Medical Services
Division for Intellectual and Developmental Disabilities
Ministry of Social Affairs and Social Services
PO Box 1260, IL-91012 Jerusalem, Israel
E-mail: jmerrick@zahav.net.il
Home-page: http://jmerrick50.googlepages.com/home

Index

I

L

M

N

P

Q

R

S